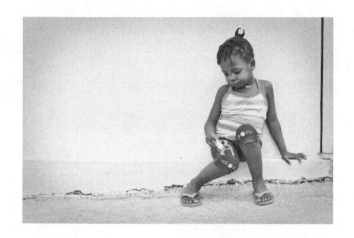

Finding Chika

Finding Chika

A little girl, an earthquake, and
the making of a family

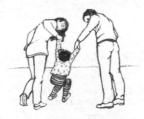

Mitch Albom

HARPER

An Imprint of HarperCollins*Publishers*

HarperCollins books may be purchased for educational, business, or sales promotional use. For information, please email the Special Markets Department at SPsales@harpercollins.com.

FIRST EDITION

All photographs are courtesy of the author except the following: Frontispiece courtesy of Jennifer Hambrick. Photograph for chapter 1 courtesy of Erika Carley. Photograph for chapter 6 courtesy of Kathleen Domish.

Grateful acknowledgment is made for permission for use of the following: "The End" from NOW WE ARE SIX by A. A. Milne, copyright 1927 by Penguin Random House LLC. Copyright © renewed 1955 by A. A. Milne. Used by permission of Dutton Children's Books, an imprint of Penguin Young Readers Group, a division of Penguin Random House LLC. All rights reserved.

Illustration by Marien Van Mechelen

Library of Congress Cataloging-in-Publication Data has been applied for.

ISBN 978-0-06-295239-4

19 20 21 22 23   LSC   10 9 8 7 6 5 4 3 2 1

To the kids at the Have Faith Haiti Orphanage, who show us, every day, the incredible resilience of children

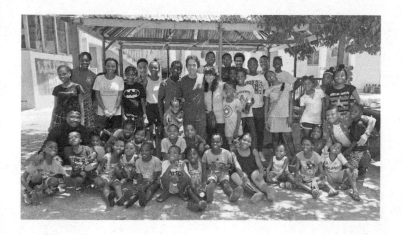

When I was One,
I had just begun.

When I was Two,
I was nearly new.

When I was Three,
I was hardly me.

When I was Four,
I was not much more.

When I was Five,
I was just alive.

But now I am Six, I'm as clever as clever,
So I think I'll be six now for ever and ever.

—A. A. MILNE

One

—

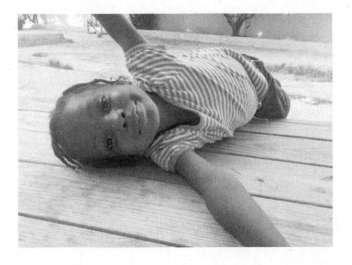

Us

———

"Why aren't you writing, Mister Mitch?"

Chika is lying on the carpet in my office. She flips onto her back. She plays with her fingers.

She comes here in the early morning, when the light is still thin at the window. Sometimes she has a doll or a set of Magic Markers. Other times, it's just her. She wears her blue pajamas, with the My Little Pony cartoon on the top and pastel stars on the bottoms. In the past, Chika loved to choose her clothes each morning after brushing her teeth, matching the colors of the socks and the shirts.

But she doesn't do that anymore.

Chika died last spring, when the trees in our yard were beginning to bud, as they are budding now, as it is spring again. Her absence left us without breath, or sleep, or appetite, and my wife and I stared straight ahead for long stretches until someone spoke to snap us out of it.

Then one morning, Chika reappeared.

"Why aren't you writing?" she says again.

My arms are crossed. I stare at the empty screen.

About what?

"About me."

I will.

"When?"

Soon.

She makes a *grrr* sound, like a cartoon tiger.

Don't be mad.

"Hmph."

Don't be mad, Chika.

"Hmph."

Don't go, OK?

She taps her little fingers on the desk, as if she has to think about it.

Chika never stays for long. She first appeared eight months after she died, the morning of my father's funeral. I walked outside to look at the sky. And suddenly, there she was, standing beside me, holding the porch railing. I said her name in disbelief—"Chika?"—and she turned, so I knew she could hear me. I spoke quickly, believing this was a dream and she would vanish at any moment.

That was then. Lately, when she appears, I am calm. I say, "Good morning, beautiful girl," and she says, "Good morning, Mister Mitch," and she sits on the floor or in her little chair, which I never removed from my office. You can get used to everything in life, I suppose. Even this.

"Why aren't you writing?" Chika repeats.

People say I should wait.

"Who?"

Friends. Colleagues.

"Why?"

I don't know.

That's a lie. I do know. *You need more time. It's too raw. You're too emotional.* Maybe they're right. Maybe when you put your loved ones down on paper, you forever accept that reality of them, and maybe I don't want to accept this reality, that Chika is gone, that words on paper are all I get.

"Watch me, Mister Mitch!"

She rolls on her back, left and right.

"The isby-bisby spider, went up a water spout . . ."

Itsy-bitsy, I correct. The words are itsy-bitsy.

"Nuh-*uhhh*," she says.

Her cheeks are full and her hair is tightly braided and her little lips pucker, as if she's going to whistle. She is the size she was when we brought her here from Haiti, as a five-year-old, and told her she was going to live with us while the doctors made her better.

"When . . .

"Will . . .

"You . . .

"Start . . .

"WRITING?"

Why does this bother you so much? I ask.

"That," she says, pointing.

I follow her finger across my desk, past souvenirs of her time with us: photos, a plastic sippy cup, her little red dragon from *Mulan*, a calendar—

"That."

The calendar? I read the date: April 6, 2018.

Tomorrow, April 7, will be one year.

One year since she left us.

Is that why you're being this way? I ask.

She looks at her feet.

"I don't want you to forget me," she mumbles.

Oh, sweetheart, I say, that's impossible. You can't forget someone you love.

She tilts her head, as if I don't know something obvious.

"Yes, you can," she says.

———

There was a night, during her first few months with us, when I read Chika *The House at Pooh Corner*. Chika loved to be read to. She would snuggle into the crook of my midsection, rest the book cover against her legs, and grab the page to turn it before I finished.

Near the end of that particular story, a departing Christopher Robin says to Pooh, "Promise you won't forget about me, ever. Not even when I'm a hundred." But the bear doesn't promise. Not at first. Instead he asks, "How old shall I be then?"—as if he wants to know what he's getting into.

It reminded me of our orphanage in Haiti and how, the moment a visitor arrives, our children ask, "How long are you staying?" as if measuring the affection they should dole out. All of them have been left behind at some point, staring at the gate, tears in their eyes, waiting for someone to return and take them home. It happened to Chika. The person who brought her departed the same day. So perhaps this is what she means. You can forget your loved ones. Or at least not come back for them.

I glance again at the calendar. Can it really be a year since she's gone? It feels like yesterday. It feels like forever.

All right, Chika, I say. I'll start writing.

"Yay!" she squeals, shaking her fists.

One condition.

She stops shaking.

You have to stay here while I do. You have to stay with me, OK?

I know she cannot do what I'm asking. Still, I bargain. It's all we really want, my wife and I, since Chika has been gone; to be in the same place with her, all the time.

"Tell me my story," Chika says.

And you'll stay?

"I'll try."

All right, I say. I will tell you the story of you and me.

"Us," she says.

Us, I say.

You

———

Once upon a time, Chika, I came to your country. I wasn't there the day you were born. I arrived a few weeks later, because a really bad thing happened. It was called an earthquake. An earthquake is when—

Us

———

"—Mister Mitch. Stop."

What's the matter?

"Don't talk like that."

Like what?

"Like I'm a baby."

But you're only seven.

"Nuh-uh."

You're not seven anymore?

She shakes her head.

How old are you?

She shrugs.

What should I do?

"Talk like a grown-up. Like you talk to Miss Janine."

You're sure?

She takes my wrists and guides them back to the keys. I feel the warmth of her little hands and I revel in it. I have learned I cannot touch Chika, but she can touch me. I am not sure why this is. I don't get the rules. But I am grateful for her visits and hungry for every little contact.

I start again.

You

———

I wasn't there the day you were born, Chika. I arrived in Haiti a few weeks later, to help after a terrible earthquake, and since you tell me I should talk like a grown-up, then I can say it was seismic enough in thirty seconds to wipe out nearly three percent of your country's population. Buildings crumbled. Offices collapsed. Houses that held families were intact one moment and puffs of smoke the next. People died and were buried in the rubble, many of them not found until weeks later, their skin covered in gray dust. They never did get an accurate count of those lost, not to this day, but it was in the hundreds of thousands. That's more people killed in less than a minute than in all the days of the American Revolution and the Gulf War combined.

It was a tragedy on an island where tragedy is no stranger. Haiti, your homeland, is the second poorest nation in the world, with a history of hardship and many deaths, the kind that come too soon.

But it is also a place of great happiness, Chika. A place of beauty and laughter and unshakable faith, and children—children who, in a rainstorm, will hook arms and dance spontaneously, then throw themselves to the ground in hysterics, as if they don't know what to do with all their joy. You were happy there in that way once, even very poor.

———

The story of your birth was told to me as follows: on January 9, 2010, you entered this world inside a two-room cinder block house by a breadfruit tree. There was no doctor present. A midwife named Albert delivered you from your mother's womb. From all accounts, yours was a healthy birth, you cried when you were supposed to, you slept when you were supposed to.

And on your third day of life, January 12, a hot afternoon, you were sleeping on your mother's chest when the world shook as if the dirt held thunder. Your cinder block house wobbled and the roof fell off and the structure split open like a walnut, leaving the two of you exposed to the heavens.

Perhaps God got a good look at you, Chika, because He didn't take you that day, and He didn't take your mother, even though He took so many others. Your home was destroyed, but you were both left intact—naked to the sky, but intact. All around, people were running and falling and praying and crying. Trees lay on their sides. Animals hid.

You slept that night in the sugarcane fields, on a bed of leaves, under the stars, and you slept there for many days that followed. So you were birthed into the soil of your homeland, Chika, all its roiling rage and beauty, and maybe that is why you sometimes roiled and raged yourself, and were so beautiful.

You are Haitian. Although you lived in America and died in America, you were always of another place, as you are now, even as you sit here with me.

Us

"That's better," Chika says, lying on her back.

Good, I say.

"Mister Mitch?"

Yes?

"I know about the *trembleman te.*"

The earthquake.

"It was bad."

Yes, it was.

"Mister Mitch?"

Yes?

"I have to tell you something."

What?

"I can't stay."

Her big eyes look up at me, and I swear, even if I were a mile away, I could still see them. They say a child's eyes are fully formed around age three, and that is why they appear so large on the face. Or maybe those years are just so full of wonder, the child can't help it.

Can I keep going? I ask. For now?

She purses her lips and shakes her head back and forth, as if she just tasted a bitter lemon. She did this all the time when she was alive, as if every thought needed a tumble through her brain.

"Keep going," she decides.

You

———

Once, late at night, Miss Janine and I were crouched next to your bed and you said to us, quietly, "How did you find me?"

I thought it such a sad question that I could only repeat it. "How did we find you?" And you said, "Yes." And we said, "You mean how did you come to us?" and you said yes, again. But I think you meant it the way you said it, because life before the orphanage was foggy in your memory, like being in a misty forest, so "How did you find me?" makes sense, because to you, I suppose, it felt as if you were found.

But you were never lost, Chika. I want you to know that. There were people who loved you before we loved you. Your mother, Resilia, from what I have been told, was a tall, strong woman with a broad face and a stern expression, like you have sometimes when you do not get your way. The daughter of a yam farmer in the seaport of Aux Cayes, she came to Port-au-Prince when she was seventeen. She liked to read and eat fish and she sold little things on the street to earn money. She had a friend named Herzulia, and they would take walks together and laugh about men and eventually your mother got involved with a man of her own, an older man with sad eyes whose first name was Fedner and whose last name was Jeune, which is your last name, too. *Jeune*, in French, means "young," so it suits you.

Your mother and Fedner had two girls who preceded you, your older sisters, and when your mother got pregnant with you, she told Herzulia that you would be her last child. Together they chose an elegant name for you, Medjerda, although very soon everyone was calling you Chika. Someone said it was because you were a stocky baby. Someone else said *Chika* is a term of endearment. It doesn't really matter. We have names we are given and names that just attach to us, and Chika was yours. And had your mother been right, had you been her last child, she might be alive and I might never have met you.

But she and Fedner had one more baby after you, two years later, a boy. He arrived in the hottest month of the year, August, in the early hours before the sun came up. Albert, the midwife, was again present, but this time something went wrong.

Your new brother lived.

Your mother died.

I know it makes no sense to have birth and death in the same bed, Chika, but that is what happened, and that was the last you saw of your birth family for a long time. Herzulia carried you off after the funeral. She said your mother had chosen her as your godmother and had insisted, "If I ever die, you must take Chika." So she did. Your father did not object. He did not keep any of his children. Maybe he was too stunned by your mother's death, and he literally did not know what to do.

Whatever the case, your oldest sister, Muriel, went with an aunt, your second oldest, Mirlanda, went with a family friend, your new baby brother, Moïse—whose namesake in the Bible was raised by an Egyptian princess—went with your mother's brother, to a cramped apartment he shared with his wife.

And you went with Herzulia, a short, strong woman with a high, thready voice who loved your mother very much and who cried the whole day of her funeral. She took you and two sets of your clothes that afternoon and together you rode off in the back of a Haitian tap-tap bus.

Those clothes were all you got to keep from your first home, Chika. It is not a lot, I know. I can only say that God was merciful by not letting you remember those days. Your mother was buried in a large grave with other people, and there is no marker for her anywhere, nothing with her name that you can visit or pray over, although you can always pray wherever you are, you know this from your teachings.

Your next home did not last long. Less than a year. It was a single-room apartment in a cinder block structure that you shared with Herzulia's family. There was no bathroom inside. At night, when the electricity went off, it was total darkness, and in the mornings, you would carry dirty bedsheets up the stairs to the rooftop, a dangerous undertaking for a child not yet three years old. A woman saw you doing this and grew concerned for your safety. She suggested to Herzulia that you might be better off in an orphanage. She knew of one not far away, in the section of the city known as Delmas 33.

That is the orphanage I have operated since 2010, the year of the earthquake, the place you called *misyon an*, "the mission," specifically, the Have Faith Haiti Mission, a rectangular piece of land behind a high gray gate on Rue Anne Laramie, a terribly potholed street that gathers water like a small lake when it rains.

And that, Chika, was the beginning of providence moving our lives together, or the continuance of it, I should say, since the Lord doesn't get ideas partway through a life.

———

Do you remember meeting me? You said sometimes you did, but other times I wondered, because you were still so young, only three. You had clips and ribbons in your hair, and you were wearing a pink dress that Herzulia picked out, because the Haitian adults who come to us often feel if their young ones are well attired, we will be more inclined to take them. This is not true, of course. At times it seems incongruous, dressing up children who are being brought to us in poverty. Perhaps it is about pride, which is something you must respect, especially in a foreign country, because you won't always understand it, and there were many times in Haiti I did not.

To be honest, Chika, for my first few years, I didn't understand a great deal about Haiti, or the orphanage, or how I was supposed to make the place work. The power would go off every day, the water would run out, deliveries of rice and bulgur would start and stop, and we never had enough medicine. Repair people would say they were on their way, then never show up. Paperwork—from receipts to government documents—was done by hand. I was a writer by trade, living in Detroit, and while I had overseen some charitable operations in America, in Haiti, I often felt like a man trying to read assembly instructions in another language.

On top of that, Miss Janine and I had no children of our own. So despite my enthusiasm, I was inexperienced with parental things. I fumbled with tiny zippers and buttons. I overreacted when a child threw up. I stumbled through explaining puberty to our boys.

But I knew this: when children were brought to our gate, I had to look past their appearances, because there were so many, and so much need, and for every child we could say yes to, even now, there are ten to whom we cannot. The majority of Haitians live on less than two dollars a day, and many have no power, no clean water, and must rely on charcoal for cooking. For every thousand babies born, eighty will die before their fifth birthday.

Keeping children safe and fed is a desperate priority for many Haitians, Chika. A place like ours can offer that hope. Perhaps that's why so many come. And when they do I must ask questions. Such as, how are the children living? How are they eating? What dire conditions have brought them to us?

You should know that when I ask such things, the adult will sometimes burst into tears. One mother in her early twenties came to us so pregnant I thought she might give birth in the office. She had a son, maybe four years old, standing beside her, and an infant in her arms. She begged us to take them both, because she had no money, no job, no home, no food to feed them. When I asked how she would provide for the baby she was carrying, she cried out, *"Ou mèt pran li tou,"* you can have it as well.

She was not being heartless. I believe that she loved her children—so much so that she wanted a safer life for them, even if it meant she could no longer see them every day. It takes a special strength to take care of a child, Chika, and a whole different strength to admit you cannot.

Perhaps Herzulia felt this when she brought you to us. She said she had three children of her own and no money. As we talked you watched in silence, Herzulia occasionally straightening your dress.

Here is what I remember the most. After a while, you crossed your arms, as if you were getting impatient, and I looked at you and you looked back, and I stuck out my tongue and you stuck out yours, and I laughed and you laughed in return.

Most new children, when brought to our mission, are shy

and nervous and look away if I catch their glance. But you went eye-to-eye with me, right from the start.

And even though I knew so little about you, Chika, I could tell that you were brave, and I knew that being brave would help you in this life.

I did not know how much.

Us

———

"Wait, Mister Mitch."

Yes?

"I have a question."

All right.

She puts her hands on my desk and pushes against it. "When I came to the mission, did I cry?"

No.

"Was I mad?"

I don't think so. Why would you be mad?

"Because I was so little!" she intones, as if it's obvious. "And I had to go away!"

Are you mad about that now?

"No." She looks off. "I don't get mad anymore."

This actually saddens me, because Chika's temper was one of her most endearing traits. She would cross her arms and turn away from us, dropping her chin deep into her chest. If I came up on her right, she'd spin left, on her left, she'd spin right. When I squatted in front of her and held her by the shoulders, I'd have to suppress a grin. Such a scowl!

Although she was just a child, Chika had perfected the look of a middle-aged man on a long bank line.

Are you happier now, I ask, not getting mad?

"Sometimes I miss it."

When?

"Like, remember if I yelled, and you and Miss Janine would tell me, 'Chika, we don't yell at each other'?"

That's when you miss being mad?

"I don't miss being *maaaad*," she drawls. "I miss you telling me *not* to be."

I pause and swallow, the way I often did during her life, when her inadvertent wisdom caught me off guard.

"Mister Mitch?"

Yes?

"Was I your favorite kid in Haiti?"

The question makes me smile. The fact is, from the day we took her in, Chika was a bossy ball of fire who was soon directing the other kids like a drill sergeant, even the older ones, telling them who should go first in relay races, which doll they should play with, where to stand on line for the bathroom. She had a strong voice and a stubborn streak, and I believe some of the shyer kids were terrified of her. I wish I knew where her bravado came from, what happened before us that made her so bold. All I know is when I look at photos from those early days, she is often posed with one hand on a jutting hip, wagging a finger, and you can almost hear her saying, "No, no, no."

You are all my favorites, I tell her now.

"You always say that."

Well, you are.

She rolls on her stomach and suddenly has a doll. I don't know where it came from. It's a princess of some kind, with a blue dress, black hair, and a tiara. She pushes both arms up, so the doll is reaching for the heavens.

"Mister Mitch?"

Umm?

"Why didn't you have babies?"

I pause.

What do you mean?

"You said people brought you their babies, but you and Miss Janine didn't have babies."

I'm writing your story, Chika. What does that have to do with your story?

Her eyelids lift like a clamshell opening. She knows it had everything to do with her story.

Me

Well. All right. The true answer is selfishness. I have always warned you about being selfish, Chika, but that does not mean I was not selfish myself. I was, often, especially when I was younger, and especially with my time. I thought there was so much left. I thought starting a family was like a new carpet I could store in a closet and unroll when I was ready.

So during my dating years, if a woman spoke too much about children, I ended things. Work was my focus, covering sports, and I took on every assignment I could get. My one long relationship, before Miss Janine, went as far as an engagement ring, but the woman changed her mind and abruptly left—to marry another man—and after a few months of hurt and confusion, I told myself maybe it was for the best.

I passed through my twenties, chasing success, and was in my early thirties when I met Miss Janine. And even though I fell deeply in love with her, I hesitated. She was beautiful and patient and saw the best in me, even when I did not deserve it. But when it came to marrying, a part of me remembered what had happened before and made me wonder: How can you be sure? Maybe something else is destined for you? I see now that was just a way to maintain Miss Janine's company without committing to a future. It was selfish, Chika, and when I finally realized how lucky I was to be with her, a lot of time had passed.

We married seven years after we met, when we were both in our late thirties. Yet even after the wedding, I delayed us starting a family, saying we should enjoy being married for a while, not rush into it. And soon, all that was left for us was to rush, and meet with doctors, and try extra things to have babies. But those things did not work, and the years passed, and soon it was impractical and even unsafe.

Eventually, we settled into different roles: aunt and uncle. Between us we had seven brothers and sisters, who between them had fifteen children. We babysat. We played. We attended our nieces' and nephews' school assemblies, took them for dinners and on vacations. On Christmas Eve, when the families gathered, we gave them all presents.

But on Christmas morning, we woke up to a silent house, and I sometimes found Miss Janine crying in our bedroom. It is all right not to have children if you don't want them, Chika, but if you do, their absence can be aching. It was my fault. To this day, it pains me. There are many kinds of selfishness in this world, but the most selfish is hoarding time, because none of us know how much we have, and it is an affront to God to assume there will be more.

Us

"Mister Mitch?"

Yes?

"Did you say you were sorry?"

To Miss Janine? Many times.

"Did she say, 'It's OK'?"

Kind of.

"Because you learned your lesson?"

What do you mean?

"That's what Miss Janine would say to me. 'Did you learn your lesson, Chika?' And if I said yes, she would say, 'Then it's OK. As long as you learned your lesson.'" She mimics my wife's voice. "'It's OK, Chika. I love you, Chika.'" Chika likes saying the word *Chika*.

I guess I learned my lesson, I say. I'm still learning new ones.

"But you are not in school!"

Not school lessons, Chika. Lessons about the world and how to live in it. You taught me some.

"Me?"

She seems genuinely surprised. She places her hands on

the sides of my face. The warmth of her fingers loosens something inside me, and despite knowing better, I blurt out the question: *How are you here?*

For a moment, she appears very serious. Then she wags her tongue and makes a *b-duh-b-duh-b-duh* noise. She laughs and releases me. The warmth departs.

"Can I have a piece of paper?" she says.

I hand her a yellow pad.

"Can I have something to draw with?"

I hand her a marker.

"Mister Mitch? Did I really teached you something?"

Teach me. Yes. You taught me many things.

"Then here!"

She slaps the pad and marker on my desk. Her voice rises. "Now I am the teacher! You have to write what I teached you! And don't stop"—she wags a parental finger—"until you are finished!"

Why?

"Because then I can stay."

Wait, I say. Forever?

But she is gone.

Two

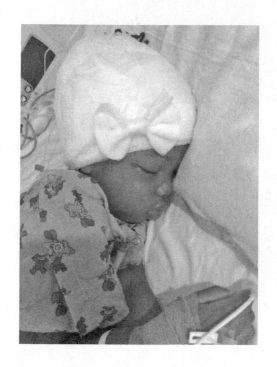

It is August of 2013. I have been operating the orphanage for three years. We have functional water, healthy food, and many new children. And while much of Haiti remains a mystery to me, coming here every month has made certain things routine.

I land at the Port-au-Prince airport, go through passport control, shuffle past a small Haitian band playing welcome music. I descend the escalator, which, per usual, is not working.

Alain Charles, our Haitian director, stands at the bottom, having talked his way inside. (By now he knows nearly everyone who works here.) We retrieve the bags and push out the doors, which is like entering a tunnel of burning air. Sweating men in button-down shirts grab at my luggage and yell, "Hello, sir! . . . I help you, sir!" We fight the crowd to reach the car.

As we weave through heavy traffic, we pass piles of earthquake rubble, still visible after three years, and mounds of trash, some of it on fire. A stray goat. A skinny dog. Potholes that could swallow a vehicle whole. Finally, with a horn honk, a security guard opens the gate of our orphanage. We pass through and honk again.

I open my door and the whole world changes.

I hear the most wonderful sound—squealing children—running my way. They are led by our newest arrival, Chika Jeune, who has only been here a few weeks. The others yell, "Mister Mitch!" but she doesn't really know me yet. Still, she seems determined to be first. The kids grab my legs and jump on my waist and she raises her arms, so I lift her up. I am often amazed by how little a child needs to know you to want your embrace.

"And how are you, Chika Jeune?"

She doesn't answer. She speaks no English.

"Sak pase?" I try, a Creole expression akin to "What's up?"

She grins and grabs my neck and buries her head.

"It's OK," I say, "you'll talk later."

Us

———

It is May before Chika visits me again. The anniversary of her passing comes and goes, and while we receive calls and sympathy cards and emails from loved ones, there is no appearance from Chika herself. Each morning I go down to my office and linger by the computer, watching old videos of her, waiting. But she does not come.

Sometimes, I take the marker she left me and slide the pad beneath it, tapping on it with the closed tip. *What she taught me.* Where would I even start? I keep thinking about what she said, that she would stay forever if I completed this task. And while I know that is impossible, I can't ignore the temptation. If I'm really going to write about her, and me, and us, maybe that's the way to do it.

So, eventually, because Chika loved numbers, I put a number down for each big lesson learned. I could list hundreds. I stop at seven.

She died on the seventh.

She was seven years old.

I wait for her return.

Finally, on a rainy Monday morning, Chika reappears. She

is sitting on the edge of my desk, her little legs dangling. I am relieved to see her, but I say only, "Good morning, beautiful girl," as I did every morning when she was alive.

"Good morning, Mister Mitch." Her voice is froggy, as if she just woke up. She lowers herself to the floor and begins poking around for the list.

I missed you, Chika.

She doesn't answer, but I can see she is pleased. Often we'd tell Chika "I missed you" or "I love you," and rather than responding, she would merely tilt her head, as if watching the words float toward her, absorbing the sentence like sunshine on her face.

"Did you write something, Mister Mitch?"

Yes.

I point to the yellow pad, and she leans over for a better look. The first line reads: "I Am Your Protection."

"What does *thaaat* mean?" she says.

It means to take care of someone, Chika. To protect against danger. You know that word. *Protection.*

"Like Aslan the lion?" she says.

She's referring to *The Chronicles of Narnia.* Aslan is supposed to be Jesus. So I may have gotten in too deep here.

Sort of, I reply. I'm making a list of what you taught me. That's the first big thing. Protection.

She crosses her arms.

"I don't get it," she says.

Lesson One

———

I AM YOUR PROTECTION

Well, let's see. Do you remember once flying so high on the mission swing set that you nearly came out of the seat, and I grabbed you and slowed your trajectory? Or when we went in the ocean, and I held you beneath your arms so your head didn't go underwater?

That's one kind of protection, Chika. It probably seemed natural to you, a grown-up stepping in to stop bad things from happening. But it was new to me. Until I got to Haiti, my protecting was directed mostly to Miss Janine, my career, and myself. I protected our health. I protected our money. I protected my books and my professional reputation. I said I had been selfish, but this was not about that. Nobody needed me. Not in that crying newborn way, when a mother and father realize it is just them, and all other interests must be pushed aside.

Miss Janine and I never went through that, not with you, and not with the other kids at the orphanage, as much as we love them. We never got to hold you when you were wet and fresh to the world, nor did we root for your first steps, or pack diaper bags and animal crackers when we traveled.

In truth, we did not meet most of you until you could already walk and talk, and in many cases had been through incredible hardships: being abandoned in the woods as an infant, which happened to one of your mission brothers, or losing parents in an earthquake or a hurricane, which brought us your four little mission sisters from the town of Jérémie—some of whom had been living beneath the muddied remains of their homes for months.

I could not protect them from those things. But I was determined to protect them from anything else, just as I was determined to protect you. I had to consider things I never thought about before, like how slippery the floors were, or how potholed the concrete was where the kids played soccer, or how to intercept tiny toys that could be swallowed, or containers of diesel fuel for the generator that might get into the wrong young hands.

In the early months, I thought if I only focused more, I could guard against anything. But like walking into a swarm of bees, the more you swat at dangers, the more of them seem to appear. As we admitted more children I worried about our building (still not earthquake-proof), our upper level (what if someone fell?), our water tanks (what if something poisonous got in them?). It was overwhelming. Gradually, I had to face the fact that I could not control everything, no matter how fast my eyes darted from spot to spot. This was hard. I am not good at being vulnerable, Chika, or relying on the Lord to handle it all, even though many around me in Haiti were at peace under His watch. Protecting our kids became the biggest and most anxious priority in my life.

But because you were all so young, I thought more about accidents and mishaps, not long-term health.

Then, one day, when I was back in Michigan, I got a phone call from Mr. Alain.

"Sir, there is something wrong with Chika."

"What's wrong?" I said.

"Her face. It is drooped. And she is walking funny."

"Did you take her to the doctor?"

"Yes, sir."

"What did he do?"

"He gave her eyedrops."

"Alain, it's not her eyes. Can you find a neurologist?"

"Sir?"

"A nerve doctor."

"I will find one."

I remember hanging up and feeling unsettled, as if something ominous was coming, like the rolling thunder on Haitian afternoons before the heavy rains fall. We never needed a neurologist before, Chika. A skin doctor, yes. A dentist, sure. Cough medicine, diarrhea medicine, children's Tylenol. But a neurologist?

How serious is this? I wondered.

———

When we finally found that neurologist, he noted the droop of your mouth and your left eye, and how your gait was slightly off. He ordered an MRI. At the time, there was only one MRI machine in Haiti, and it cost $750 cash for an appointment.

Mr. Alain took you there. You left before sunrise. Six hours later, a nurse finally called your name. She made you drink a syrup that put you to sleep. You were placed inside a large cylinder, where radio waves and a magnetic field were generated around your head. The results were images that showed you from the inside.

And while I would have told people that on the inside, Chika, you were warm and curious and confident and funny, the MRI analysis was more clinical:

"The child has a mass on her brain. We don't know what it is. But whatever it is, there is no one in Haiti who can help her."

I read that.

And everything I knew about protection changed.

Us

———

"Mister Mitch?"

Yes?

"The drink was sweet."

What drink?

"The drink the nurse gave me. It made me sleepy."

That's why you drank it.

"But I woke up."

In the machine?

"Yeah. I started crying."

You woke up inside the MRI machine? Then what happened?

"They made me drink more. And I fell asleep again."

I shake my head. It is folly to compare America's medical care system to Haiti's. The challenges for doctors and nurses are almost unimaginable, the poverty, the malnutrition, patients' lack of access to health care or education. Still, I recall being struck by the bluntness of Chika's MRI report: *Whatever it is, there is no one in Haiti who can help her.* It seemed less a diagnosis than a surrender.

"Mister Mitch?"

Yes?

She leans against my leg. I instinctively reach to hold her shoulders, but my fingers pass right through. The rules of engagement. I keep forgetting.

"Tell me about when I came to America," she says.

You

———

All right. Here is what I recall. You were the first child we ever brought to this country, and the day of your departure, the other kids at the mission lined up to hug you. They waved goodbye as the car left the gates. I imagine some thought they would never see you again.

Accompanied by Mr. Alain, you flew to Miami and on to Detroit, wearing a white sweater, even though it was June. In your first American bathroom, you turned the faucet and jerked your hands back, because you had never felt hot water from a sink before. So before you even slept a night here, this country was a wonder to you.

Miss Janine and I were waiting at the house, and Miss Janine had arranged some colorful blankets and dolls to make you feel welcome. At the time, we hoped the doctors would diagnose the problem and treat it quickly, and you would heal under our watch. Then you could return to Haiti. We thought this would take a few months. Looking back now, we really knew so little.

I should say you did not seem scared when you got here, Chika, but you did not speak much, either. Or show much emotion. Mostly you looked around. Who could blame you? Virtually everything you saw was new: traffic lights, highways, houses with yards, mailboxes, televisions in different rooms. The input had to be overwhelming. I often wondered, when you went to sleep that first night, how far you imagined yourself from the mission.

The day after your arrival, we went for tests at Mott Children's Hospital in Ann Arbor, part of the University of Michigan, a great school that I'd dreamed you and the other children might one day attend. It was the tallest building you had ever seen, and you gazed up as we walked inside. We approached the front desk. A man said hello. He gave you a wristband, which you admired like a bracelet.

Then the man turned to me and asked, "What is your relationship to the patient?"

For a moment, I hesitated. All around were mothers and fathers, many looking similar to their children, same hair, same skin color, same facial features. I felt as if I'd been caught trying to fool someone. I answered by saying "legal guardian," because those are technically the correct words, and the man wrote something down and asked me to stand before a camera.

"Mister Mitch!" you suddenly yelled. "Look!" You pointed to a large Superman figure in the lobby. I released your hand and you ran to it, just as the man handed me a sticker with a grainy photo of my face.

Above the photo was one word: *Parent.*

I stuck it to my shirt.

It is the fall of 2013, and Chika Jeune has been at our orphanage for a few months. As the smallest and youngest, she goes first in line for the bathrooms, or for school. She seems to enjoy the other kids marching behind her. Still, I often see her playing by herself, preferring to take a toy to a private corner. New children are frequently quiet, finding a coloring book or a doll to cling to, perhaps because there's nothing to cling to from their past. I wonder how long it will take Chika to move from outsider to insider.

One evening, we are doing our nightly devotions, a tradition of prayers and effusive gospel singing, punctuated by bongo drums and energized by the sheer volume of high-pitched voices. The kids will yell out a song and launch into it, some in Creole, some in English, from "Shout to the Lord" and "I Give Myself Away" to "Jeriko Miray-La Kraze" and "Mwen se Solda Jezi." Sometimes, it sounds like screaming in a sports rally. But it remains a sight to behold, young ones with so little, singing their thanks to the Lord.

On this night I am sitting by a wall, with several kids leaning against me. In the middle of an upbeat song, Janine catches my attention.

"Look," she says, pointing.

There, a few feet away, is Chika Jeune, in a white nightshirt, clapping and swaying her head to the beat. Her eyes are closed, and she is punching the air and laughing between the lyrics. When the song ends, she throws an arm over her braided hair and gives the sweetest openmouthed smile, as if to say, "That was fun. Can we do it again?"

I make a mental note. The praying did it. She's in.

Me

———

I guess I should explain, Chika, what I was doing in Haiti when you came to us, and how I wound up in charge of an orphanage seventeen hundred miles from home.

It began, as many good things do, with a coincidence.

A few days after the earthquake, a local pastor named John Hearn Jr. came on a radio show I host in Detroit. He was worried that a Port-au-Prince mission he was associated with had been destroyed, and that the children there might have died. He could not get a phone call through (few people could at the time) and he was seeking help.

His story moved me greatly. I'm not sure why. In my role as a journalist, I have interviewed many people after natural disasters. And while I have always encouraged assistance, I've rarely provided it personally.

This was different. Something about not knowing the fate of children seemed terrifying. I tried to organize a trip for the pastor, but there were still, at that time, no commercial flights going into Haiti. I was finally able to charter a small plane and found two pilots willing to fly it. The plane held six passengers, so Hearn brought along his father, John, who had helped start the mission, and an elderly woman named Florence "Mommy" Moffett, a quiet, lovely missionary who had lived and worked at the orphanage for years. I recruited two colleagues who filled the other seats.

And with the help of a U.S. senator named Carl Levin, we were granted—by the American military, which was controlling air traffic into Haiti after the earthquake—a ten-minute window to land. We took off from the snow in Pontiac, Michigan.

Nearly five hours later, we descended into the heat-baked runways of the Port-au-Prince airport, or what was left of it.

When the engines shut off, I left my winter coat on the seat and stepped outside. The sun was intense. The air was still. In the distance were mountains and more mountains ("land of high mountains" is the aboriginal meaning of the word *Haiti*). Mostly it was quiet. Eerily quiet, as if the country were mired in a stunned aftershock. I studied the facade of the sand-colored terminal. It read: AEROPORT INTERNATIONAL TOUSSAINT LOUVERTURE, named for the leader of the Haitian revolution more than two centuries ago.

Thanks to the earthquake, there was now a large crack over the word *Toussaint*.

We unloaded the cargo with no officials, and no security. The only nod to a functioning airport was in a terminal hallway, where a fold-up table had several women sitting behind it, beneath a piece of white paper taped to the wall. It read:

"STOP!!! HAITI IMMIGRATION."

We passed through in a minute.

The ride to the orphanage, in a wobbly blue van miss-ing its door panel, was only twenty minutes, but it will be etched in my mind forever: street after street of what used to be buildings, now flattened, their insides spilled out in mountains of gray rubble, as if fed through a blender. The chunky piles were spiked by the occasional leg of a desk, or a mattress. Crushed cars were abandoned under debris. People wandered the streets like zombies. Grim-faced street vendors squatted near piles of clothing, and women hovered over rotted fruits and vegetables. Kids stood in line to gather water from street puddles.

Everyone appeared to be outside. I saw nobody in a win-dow or coming out a door. I would later learn that many Haitians refused to enter buildings for months, fearful that the remaining structures would collapse on top of them. The choked air smelled of diesel and burning trash, and my eyes were stinging before we even reached our destination.

The orphanage itself was, thankfully, spared. But it was overrun with outsiders, who mixed with children in make-shift tents. In Haiti, after natural disasters, people often flock to orphanages and hospitals, believing relief agencies will bring food there first. But I saw little in the way of relief or food, outside of some rice and beans cooked over charcoal by women I presumed to be orphanage staff.

It was impossible to tell who belonged there and who had wandered in. Laundry lines crisscrossed the yard, old foam mattresses were scattered on the dirt. There were many weary-looking people, leaning against the walls, squinting into the sun. They asked for food. When we opened the boxes that we'd crammed on the plane—bottled water, Sani-Cloth Wipes, jars of aspirin, cans of Coke—we were mobbed.

At one point, I became dazed by all that I was seeing. It was steamy hot and my shirt was soaked and I was foolishly wearing black jeans, which imprisoned the heat against my legs. I exhaled hard.

And suddenly, with my arms by my side, I felt two little hands slip into my fingers. I glanced down to see a little boy and girl, one on each side. I can't tell you who they were, Chika, or even if they belonged at the orphanage. But they smiled and led me forward, and I realize now they were walking me into their world and, in time, into yours.

But all right. I haven't explained how a trip turned into a commitment. Upon returning to Detroit, I wrote about what I'd seen and asked for help. We quickly organized a team of volunteers: roofers, plumbers, electricians, contractors. There were twenty-three of them in all, and they dubbed themselves The Detroit Muscle Crew. With airplanes donated by Roger Penske, the former race car driver turned successful businessman, and Art Van Elslander, owner of the Art Van furniture chain, we packed up with supplies, tools, and small machinery and headed back to Port-au-Prince.

Then we went again.

And again.

And again.

Over nine separate trips, alongside Haitian laborers, we built toilets, a kitchen, a dining room, and a laundry area. We laid tile. We assembled bunk beds. We painted filthy walls with bright sherbet colors. We eventually constructed a three-room school.

We also built the orphanage's first showers, jerry-rigged with white PVC pipe that ran down from a rooftop water tank. To that point, the kids' bathing had been limited to soapy water dumped from a large red bucket.

When time came to test those showers, the youngest children crowded inside. Wearing shorts or underwear, they stared curiously at the knobs and the faucet. We counted "one, two, three" and opened the pressure. The water sprayed down and they howled in delight, as if experiencing the Lord's first rainstorm. They splashed and laughed and sang and did a dance. They were so joyous, doing something I all but sleepwalked through every morning of my life, that my heart shifted. I could physically feel it, an epiphany maybe, because that word means the manifestation of something divine, and that is how it felt, and how the following days there felt. I was exhausted yet elevated in an almost unearthly way. I found myself laughing more freely than I did in the States, and sleeping better. Each day I felt less encumbered, despite a workload that began at sunrise and ended in mosquito-swarmed darkness.

"I think we can make a difference here," I told Miss Janine.

"Then we should keep going," she said.

And we did. I flew down every month. In America, my daily life was a good deal about thinking—creating stories, making decisions, adjusting my schedule, juggling phone calls. In Haiti, there were just *things to do,* and what we did allowed children to eat, to sleep, to have shelter; things so primary, there was no debating their importance. With each visit my connection to the kids grew stronger. I learned their names and personalities. I was greeted by their leaping embraces. It was adults who brought me to Haiti, Chika, but it was children that brought me back.

In Detroit, I met again with the senior John Hearn, who was in his mid-eighties. He explained his history with the place. Over time, he said, the burden had increased. He thanked me for all the physical improvements our Muscle Crew was making. But he admitted he didn't have the money to operate the orphanage, and hadn't in some time. He himself was only able to go down there periodically.

Which is when, in a rush of something I cannot to this day explain, I referenced other charities I had created in Detroit and blurted out, "If you want, I could take over running the orphanage. I can find the money. And the people. I think."

He clasped his hands together and grinned.

We signed papers.

And I have been there ever s—

Us

———

—"OK, OK, OK," Chika interrupts, sighing.

OK what?

She lifts one of my coffee cups.

"Too much talking about you!"

She plops the cup down.

"I wanna hear about ME!"

My instinct is to remind her about manners, but I don't. I have always found something forgivable about children seeking attention and the lengths they will go to get it. Chika liked center court. If Janine and I would speak too long, she'd yell, "Hey, what are you guys *talking* about?" If we sat to play a board game, she'd grab the pieces and instruct, "You are the green. I am the red. Red is the boss!"

Of course, when she first arrived, her English was more limited, so we navigated through sentences like "Help, I not can open" when she was holding a banana, or, "There is him!" if she spotted a lost toy. Pronouns took a long time.

But as the weeks passed, and Chika added sentence after sentence, we witnessed an exceptional development, and a boundless curiosity about her past and future.

"When will I fall in love?" she asked us one night.

Janine and I just looked at each other.

"Well, when you're older," Janine finally said. "And you meet the right person."

"But when will *that* be?"

"We don't know."

"Why do you want to fall in love, Chika?" I asked.

She made a face. "Because *you* fell in love"—she crossed her arms—"and *I* wanna fall in love!"

She said it so emphatically, I half expected the Lord to produce someone for her right then and there.

"And who do you want to fall in love with?" I asked.

"I don't know," she replied. "I want to fall in love with someone I never *met* before!"

"Why?"

"Because that's how *you* did it. You fell in love with Miss Janine. And you haven't *met* her before!"

I was left speechless at how her mind worked. But my heart was full. In a way, she was saying she wanted a love like ours. It made us feel like we were doing something right.

"Mister Mitch?" Chika says now.

Hmm?

She puts back the coffee cup and pushes two hands against my knee. Then she looks me in the eye. And the one thing she's never asked me before, she finally asks.

"How did I get sick?"

You

Well.

How do I explain this?

The Creole word for "head" is *tèt*. You know that, of course. Haitians use it in many expressions. Like *tèt vire* (a spinning head), which means "dizzy," or *tèt ansanm* (heads together), which means "unity," or *tèt frèt* (cold head), which means "calm."

Or *tèt chaje* (loaded head), which means "trouble."

You might never have learned that last one, Chika, but it fits your story, because most every part of you was perfect when you came to us, your lungs, your tummy, your heart, but just above your neck, in the part of the brain they call the pons, you were *tèt chaje*, a head loaded with something. And that something would indeed prove troubling.

That first day in Ann Arbor, they took another MRI. This time there was no syrup or long wait time. We rode an elevator down to a brightly lit, antiseptic room, and they slid you inside a giant cylinder and played music through speakers. We were home in time for supper.

But when the results came back, the doctors saw the same

thing as the Haitian neurologist: an invader had squatted in your brain, a spot on the scan that was sizeable, if diffused. It was something that was not supposed to be there, on that they agreed, and the idea was to take it out. But they debated as to whether it was worth the risk.

Days passed. Finally, the doctors on a "tumor board" met and took a vote, because, much like our decision making at the orphanage, they have to be realistic with the people who come to them. Five of the eight voted yes, which meant proceed with your surgery. I tried not to think about the three who voted no.

We wanted to prepare you for what was going to happen. But your English back then wasn't what it became, and my Creole was just so-so, and anyhow Miss Janine and I decided that this was not going to be a crash course for you in brain surgery, the way it had to be for us. Maybe we made the right decision, maybe we did not. I think we did. You were five years old, and we wanted you to enjoy being five years old, so we weren't showing you drawings of lobes and ventricles.

When we woke you early on the day of the operation, we hugged and kissed you as we always did, and we sang a good morning song as you dressed in the predawn darkness. We told you we were going to the building with the Superman, where the doctors were going to help you feel better. You yawned. You chose a doll for the ride. I lifted you into the car seat.

And exactly five years, five months, and six days after you entered this world in that cinder block house by the breadfruit tree, you entered the towering Mott Children's Hospital, where they assigned us a room and brought you a gown, light blue, with dancing bears all over it. Miss Janine helped you change.

At one point, I was asked to sign consent papers in the hallway. There were diagrams, explanations. I mostly remember the part about "risk." Risk of blood clotting. Risk of transfusions. Risk of possible side effects, including "death." I tried to move through these briskly, telling myself they were required but highly unlikely warnings, the omnipresent slight chance of rain on a sunny day.

Two hours later, you were in an operating room, under anesthesia. Instruments were prepped. Doctors and nurses surrounded you. Finally, a neurosurgeon named Hugh Garton, a thin, fit man who likes to climb mountains in his spare time, opened your precious little head and witnessed the invader firsthand.

He spent a long time attacking it and trying to remove it, hours, really, a little here, a little more there, but it was entangled with so many important parts of your brain that he could not take out much; it was like that game Operation that the kids play at the mission, where if you touch the edge, you set off the buzzer.

Dr. Garton removed about ten percent of the mass and then, choosing caution, stopped there. They stitched you back up and wheeled you to the recovery area.

All this time, Miss Janine and I waited in the massive lobby, with a beeper that lit with periodic updates. Every new message sprung us forward.

Finally, in the late afternoon, it flashed SURGERY COMPLETE. An hour later, we got our first look at you. You were sleeping on your side, so small, you only took up half the gurney, with tubes and wires attached to your body, and a large white bandage with a tiny bow wrapped around your head.

My heart sank.

Of all the hospital moments we would go through together, Chika, that one was perhaps the hardest, because until that point, despite the MRIs, the consultations, even signing those consent papers, I still had not faced the full gravity of your situation. You were playful in your first days with us, chasing me around the house, and I let myself get lost in that.

Now here you were, so tiny on that gurney, knocked out by the anesthesia, surrounded by monitors. They had cut you open and worked for hours, yet nobody was saying "We got it all." There was no relief, just more questions, and days to wait before the pathology came back. They said you would be in pain for some time, and even with the drugs, we should expect some challenges.

I stared straight ahead. *I had let them do this. I had given my OK.* The thought that my decisions had in any way hurt you turned my stomach into knots.

It also left me humbled, Chika. This might be hard to understand. But to that point, I still felt, foolishly, that I was in control of things—with you, with our kids—like I was Superman in that lobby. I had strength, I had resources. If I didn't know something, I could learn it and still lead. Our kids were small. I was the grown-up. I could take care of whatever came our way.

Standing over you that day, facing the first serious medical issue in the five years I'd been operating the orphanage, that sense of control was obliterated. A sense of foreboding took its place. You were smaller than me, yes. But what if this challenge was bigger than both of us?

"Happy New Year!"

We are on the cusp of 2014, and the kids jump around and sing "Auld Lang Syne," which I taught them, minus the words, because I don't know the words. So we all just holler, "Da-daaa, da-da-da, da, da-daaaa. . . ."

It's been our tradition since my first winter at the mission. Each December 31, we have a special dinner of pizzas from a Port-au-Prince hotel, and cups of apple juice, and a large sheet cake with chocolate icing. This is followed by the lighting of sparklers, one per child. We put them in the dirt along our wall and make a wish. When the last of the sparklers burns out, it is officially "our" New Year, even though it is barely eight-thirty.

"Happy New Year, Chika," I say, kneeling beside Chika Jeune, who has been with us for about six months. "Can you say 'Happy New Year'?"

She has a solid row of baby teeth, her two front ones touching.

"'appy new year," she says.

"You know what? Tomorrow is January, which means your birthday is coming up. And you'll get to wear the birthday crown."

Her eyes widen.

"When my birt'day?" she asks.

"Nine more days."

"How old I be?"

"Four."

She considers this, and I count on my fingers to show her. When I reach four, I tap her soft cheeks and say, "Boink." She rushes forward in a happy hug, although I don't know if it's for me or for the news that she will soon be older.

Us

———

"Mister Mitch?"

Hmm?

"Then what happened?"

Hmm?

"At the hospital?"

I realize I have drifted off and am staring out the window at a dawn redwood tree, whose yellow needles are thick in these summer months. It's the only yellow tree in our backyard, and I was trying to remember if we planted it, or if it was here when we bought the house twenty-five years ago.

"Never miiiind," Chika says, waving a hand.

No, it's OK, I say. You asked. I should tell you. I just don't like this part.

"How come?"

Because it was bad news.

"Nuh-uh."

It wasn't bad news?

She shakes her head no.

———

How could she determine that? I never told her this story, the moment Janine and I entered a small consultation room a few days after Chika's surgery.

Anyone who has sat through that slice of time, when you don't know something awful and then you do, will confirm that it is literally a bend in your life, and what is critical is what you choose next; because you can view a diagnosis many ways—as a curse, a challenge, a resignation, a test from God.

Janine and I had been hopeful that morning, based on doctors' earlier analysis, that the mass in Chika's brain could be manageable. It was fuzzy on the scans. And the frozen samples they removed during surgery were not overly alarming. The hope was for a grade one tumor, most easily dealt with, but we were braced for a grade two, which they warned could involve some radiation and long-term surveillance.

Instead, Dr. Garton came into that consultation room, sat down, and, in a soft but direct voice, said the news was not good, worse than they'd thought, that Chika had something called diffuse intrinsic pontine glioma, or DIPG. When I asked if that was a grade one or two, he said it was "a four."

A four?

He began to lay out options, which included radiation therapy and experimental medications, but all I heard was "four." *Four?* I felt like I was stumbling, even as I was sitting down. *Four?* I kept listening for the part where the surgeons go back and take the whole monster out, but it never came. Apparently, if they did that, there would be nothing left of Chika's brain to function.

Four?

"I'm really sorry to be bringing you this news," Dr. Garton said. He shared some ominous truths about DIPG: There were only around three hundred cases in the United States every year; it usually struck children Chika's age, between five and nine; it quickly debilitated them—their walking, their mobility, their swallowing. And the kicker: its long-term survival rate was, basically, zero.

We were stunned. As Dr. Garton ran through the options, I remember deliberately closing my mouth, because it was hanging open, and realizing there was even more to this moment than the feeling of a piano crashing on your head; we were supposed to *make a decision*. That's why he was telling us all this horrible information.

A decision? On Chika's life? She had just gotten to America, what, a few weeks ago? We were buying her shoes. Asking if she liked scrambled eggs. She was supposed to stay a couple of months, then return to the orphanage, cured by our amazing American medicine. A decision on her life?

Janine and I exchanged glances.

"What if she were your child?" I mumbled, falling back on that shell game of putting the onus on the doctor.

"Well," Dr. Garton said, exhaling, "I would probably take her back to Haiti, let her enjoy the summer, be with her friends, until . . ."

It's in the "until" that everything awful lies.

I could see Janine tearing up. I felt my insides welling. I blurted out the question before I lost the courage to ask it.

"How long does she have?"

"Maybe four months," he said, softly, then added, "maybe five," although I think he just said five to ease the blow of four. *Four. Again, a four.* He said radiation could extend that time frame, maybe double it, although her "quality of life" might be affected, and he personally wouldn't choose it, because she'd have to stay here instead of returning home, and, in the end, it would not make a difference.

Now, generally, I am inclined to heed doctors' advice. I respect their knowledge and expertise. But when he said "quality of life," something turned in me like a crank. Here we were, sitting in America, in an extraordinary hospital in a very affluent city. "Quality of life," as we knew it, had little connection to the land in which Chika was born, and whose toughness she carried in her veins. Remembering that she'd survived an earthquake in her first days on Earth, and slept in the sugarcane fields, and endured the death of a mother she barely knew, and had already bounced between four different homes, the idea of sending her back to wait for her demise seemed cruel. I found myself growing defensive, like a manager whose boxer was being underestimated.

"She's a fighter," I finally said, looking over at Janine, who nodded. "And if she fights, we're gonna fight."

Dr. Garton leaned back. "All right," he said.

And then, for a few moments, we all just sat there, staring at an invisible battle plan.

———

"Yay!"

Chika claps her hands.

What? I say.

I realize I have been talking out loud, telling her the tale I didn't want to tell her.

"Yay!" she says again.

Why are you clapping? Because I told you the story?

No answer.

Because we chose to fight?

No answer.

Why, Chika?

She stands and takes my hands. She mashes them together.

"Clap for us, Mister Mitch!"

I flip my palms, confused.

And she is gone again.

Three

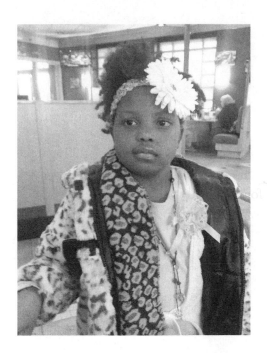

Me

——

Twenty years before Chika came to live with us, I embarked on the journey of my life. It wasn't a great distance, less than seven hundred miles on an airplane from Detroit to Boston, and a thirty-minute rental car ride to the suburb of West Newton. I had come to visit an old college professor.

His name was Morrie Schwartz.

Morrie was dying. He'd been hit with amyotrophic lateral sclerosis, ALS, the progressive neurodegenerative disorder also known as Lou Gehrig's disease, named for the famous 1930s baseball player who, forced to retire due to this illness, still announced in his farewell at Yankee Stadium, *"Today . . . I consider myself . . . the luckiest man . . . on the face of the earth."*

"Yeah. Well," Morrie would tell me, "I didn't say that."

At the time, I was thirty-seven and working five jobs, newspapers, TV, radio, books, freelance. I never said no to anything for fear I wouldn't be asked again. I only learned of Morrie's illness from television, an interview he did on ABC's *Nightline* program. Ted Koppel, the show's anchor, had flown up from Washington, D.C., to meet the elfish, dying professor, who was teaching visitors, often with a smile, what imminent death revealed about life. Koppel was so impressed with Morrie's attitude, despite no longer being able to walk, dress, or bathe on his own, that *Nightline* did an entire show on him, and would do two more.

I saw the first of these, and my jaw dropped. Morrie—a healthier version—had been my favorite college professor at Brandeis University. He taught sociology. I took every class he offered. He felt more like an uncle than a teacher. We'd walk around campus together, eat lunches together. Morrie was so ablaze with ideas, even with his mouth full, that when he spoke, little pieces of egg salad would come flying my way. (I once wrote that I had two urges the whole time I knew him: to hug him, and to hand him a napkin.)

On graduation day, I gave Morrie a present, a briefcase with his initials on it. He teared up and hugged me and said, "Mitch, you're one of the good ones. Promise me you'll stay in touch."

I promised that I would.

Then I broke that promise.

For sixteen years.

Sixteen years without a visit, a letter, even a phone call. I had no excuse except the one we all use. I was "busy"—in every pathetic way we employ that word—an in-demand sports journalist, climbing ladders, stacking successes, ever so importantly engaged, I thought.

So when I saw Morrie on *Nightline* all those years later, my shock was followed by something gnawing. Guilt. Or maybe shame. The sense that I was no longer "one of the good ones."

I called him up. I made plans to see him. It was supposed to be a single visit. But Morrie broke through something during that first encounter. Even though weak and confined to a wheelchair, he so deftly dissected me—saying, "Dying is only one thing to be sad about, Mitch. Living unhappily is something else"—that I found myself coming back, another Tuesday and another Tuesday and all the Tuesdays he had left in his life. We took one last "class" together about what truly matters in life once you know you are dying, and he pulled out of me a better, previous version of myself.

Our visits were eventually chronicled in a manuscript I wrote to pay his medical bills, *Tuesdays with Morrie,* which was supposed to be a small book yet somehow became a big book. And I became, as the years passed, an eternal graduate assistant for Morrie's final course.

It changed me. It couldn't help but change me. My conversations with strangers went from who was going to win the Super Bowl to "My mother just died and the last thing we did was read your book together. Can I talk to you about her?" Perhaps my old professor knew that my hard head would require daily knocks to reach a softer, wiser center. *Tuesdays with Morrie* provided the pounding. It was a constant riptide back into Morrie's waters, quoting him, recalling him, answering questions about him, until the actions once steered by him felt natural to me.

I was asked to speak at hospice events, medical conventions, universities. I began to visit and even counsel newly diagnosed ALS patients.

With the terminally ill, I shared Morrie's observation that his last months proved his most vibrant; he likened them to the vivid colors of a dying leaf.

With the healthy, I repeated Morrie's mantra of pretending each day to have a bird on your shoulder, a bird that you ask, "Is today the day I die?"—and to live each day as if the answer were "Yes."

So you might think the journey of my life, twenty years earlier, was part of the Lord's brilliant plan for handling Chika's prognosis, arming me with a sturdy philosophy, and a heart steeled for the grimmest of news.

Except an old man looking back on his years is not a little girl looking forward to hers.

And, as it turns out, you can have more than one journey of your life.

Us

—

Chika? I say.

I don't see her. But I hear muffled laughter.

I get out of my chair. I walk around the room. It is early September, more than a month since her last visit.

Where is Chika? I say.

This was a frequent game we played. Finding Chika. She would hide when she heard the front door open, under a blanket or beneath the kitchen table, and you'd have to yell, "Where is Chika? We lost her! Where is she?" until your voice displayed enough panic that she would burst forth and shout in her budding English, "Here is me!" Then she'd crack up laughing and throw her shoulders forward in hysterics. I have never witnessed a child happier to be discovered.

Now, apparently, we are playing the game again.

Where is Chika? I intone. Where did she go?

I see a blanket spread over a futon, which I sleep on sometimes when I write into the night. I grab the blanket. I make my voice playful.

Is she under . . . *here*? I say, yanking it up.

"Nooooo," she answers, from across the room.

I turn. She is standing by my desk, reading the yellow pad. So I guess the game is over.

"What does it mean?" she asks. "'Time Changes'?"

It's the second thing you taught me, I say. The second lesson on the list you wanted me to make.

She pulls out my chair.

"Write it."

Then she plops in the seat and laughs.

I have to sit there to write, you know.

"I know," she says and laughs again.

She spins the chair back and forth on its swivel. "*Wrrrrr! Wrrrrr!*" Suddenly, the blanket from the futon is in her hands. She pulls it over her head.

"Where is Chika?" she yells.

I sigh.

Lesson Two

———•———

TIME CHANGES

Do you remember the first morning you woke up at our house? I was already down in my office, because mornings are when I write. Suddenly, my phone rang; it was Miss Janine, calling from the bedroom. In a raspy, just-woke-up voice, she said, "Mister Mitch, Chika is hungry for breakfast. Can you help her?"

I came upstairs and led you to the kitchen, and we found eggs and butter and some cheese and tomatoes. I showed you the frying pan, the burner, and you stood on your tiptoes and helped move the spatula around. I poured juice. We said our prayers.

And I watched you eat.

And I watched you eat some more.

To call it "leisurely" doesn't come close. You chewed. You looked out the window. You put down your fork, yawned, and picked up your fork again. You swayed back and forth to some internal rhythm. It took nearly an hour. I would compare this to the pace that I eat breakfast, except I don't eat breakfast.

But the next morning, when I heard your feet thumping down the steps at 7:00 a.m., I rose from my desk, met you at the door, lifted you as you said, "Mister Mitch, I am hungry!" and carried you up to the kitchen.

A child is both an anchor and a set of wings.

My old way of doing things was gone.

Time changes. With a little one, it is no longer your own. All parents will tell you this. But perhaps because it happened to Miss Janine and me so late in life—after twenty-seven years of it being just the two of us—the difference was jolting.

When we decided you were not going back to Haiti, Chika, not until we found a way to beat this awful thing, we brought you home from the hospital with two stuffed animals, a bandage on your neck, and a suitcase full of hopeful naivete. We didn't realize the scope of this undertaking, that we were ushering in not only a child but a challenge—a full-time search for a cure to an aggressive disease that, two weeks earlier, we had barely heard of.

You had a pace. The disease had a pace. And from that point forward, all we knew about time would change, from the way we used to spend it, to the way we cherished it.

———

Do you know how old I am, Chika? You used to guess "Thirty!" and when I said no, you tried "A hundred!" Relative age must be so mysterious to children, who count their time in half years. (*"I'm five and a half!"*) But we were in our late fifties when you came to live with us, young enough to maintain our routines, old enough to bristle at changing them.

Not surprisingly, Miss Janine was faster at adapting than me. I think she was always, in some manner, preparing for this day.

On the other hand, when I was younger, I was afraid of becoming a father. I saw how it ate up the hours. I worried that I wouldn't give it the proper time and would wind up being a bad dad. Also, to be totally honest, I thought it would hinder my career. I was advancing fast and wanted to keep up that pace. Ambition is not something I ever warned you about, Chika, but I have learned it can overtake you gradually, like clouds moving across the sun, until, consumed by pursuing it, you get used to a dimmer existence.

When Miss Janine and I married, she knew all this. But she believed in a better version of me, a more generous one, and in our early years together, I wanted to live up to that. Still, hoarding time becomes a habit. I remember once, when we were trying to have children, I raised the idea of hiring an au pair to help take care of them. Miss Janine rejected it. She got angry, actually, which she rarely did. I wondered why she wouldn't welcome the help, blind to the hurt that her husband was already planning time away from a baby we didn't have.

I was a foolish man in many ways, Chika, when I look back on things.

And then you, with your unhurried ways. You were five years old, but such a curious five-year-old, as if the pages of your life had been stacked but not yet turned. If you saw squirrels darting up a tree, you shouted "Squirrels!" then asked where they were going, then asked if they could see you. You had questions about books. Questions about food. Questions about clouds and angels. You examined your entire inventory of clothes before getting dressed.

"Those red socks are good," I'd suggest, growing impatient.

"I think I want the green ones."

"The green ones are good."

"No, wait, wait. The blue."

With little choice, we slowed to your rhythm. We kneeled to your sight line. I often found you sitting on the floor by our back window, just studying the yard. I remember Morrie, my old professor, pointing to a window once and saying he appreciated it more than I did, because, due to his sickness, that window was his view of the world, while to me it was a pane of glass.

You appreciated a window more than I did, too, Chika, and all the amazing things on the other side of it. I had to decelerate to match your awe, to hit the brakes in my life, to beg out of dinners because of your bedtime, to be late for work because of places I needed to take you, to constantly apologize to bosses and editors for my suddenly slower production.

But I did. Miss Janine did, too. And we found ourselves studying you in a growing fascination. We'd nudge each other as you clapped for a movie, or danced around the table without knowing we were watching. If you nodded off in my arms, I'd hold you for a long time while Miss Janine stroked your hair. I don't know how many hours we spent just looking at you, Chika, but there were many, and they were treasured.

Before you came to us, we would watch TV in bed, and often fall asleep with the TV still playing. Once you arrived, we shut the lights and tiptoed around you in the darkness. Often, in the dead of night, you would wake us up.

"Mister Miiiitch?"

. . . "Hmm?"

"I have to go potty."

I would guide you to the bathroom, then wait, yawning, outside the doorframe. I'd hear you flush, help you wash your hands, then guide you to your bed, which was nice and low so you could tumble into it.

"Is she OK?" Miss Janine would whisper as I crawled back in beside her.

"She's fine," I'd mumble, closing my eyes. "She's good."

The most precious thing you can give someone is your time, Chika, because you can never get it back. When you don't think about getting it back, you've given it in love.

I learned that from you.

———

By the way. About your bed. It may sound funny, but when you first arrived, we didn't know where to put you. It wasn't like we'd had months to plan. Our house, which we had lived in for nearly twenty-five years, was as set in its form as we were. The guest bedrooms were downstairs. We couldn't have you that far from us. But you were too big to put in a crib.

In the end, we got a full-sized air mattress, draped it in *Frozen* sheets and colorful blankets, and set it at the foot of our bed. The first night you spent with us, I forgot it was there. I got up to use the bathroom, tripped, and went stumbling to the floor.

Eventually I got used to it. I'd remind myself in the darkness to take four extra steps before turning left, and reverse my field on the journey back. I also made a habit of leaning over you in each direction, checking on your small form, splayed between pillows, your soft breathing so different from mine.

Do you remember the day I came home to find you and Miss Janine laughing mischievously? And Miss Janine said,

"Chika, how does Mister Mitch sound when he sleeps?" And you made a loud snoring noise that suggested a lion coughing up a hairball? And I grinned stupidly and said, "Great, now there's a second set of ears on me."

Well, of course, that was true. A second set of ears, a second set of eyes and arms and legs, a second bed that we had to walk around. This is what changes hand in hand with time:

Space.

Before you, Chika, we were a pair. Now, we were a trio. Our car went from a married couple in the front seat to you and Miss Janine in the back, and me behind the wheel like a chauffeur. Tables for two became a four-top and a decision: Which of us sat next to you and helped cut your food? We expanded in every way—and it quickly became the norm.

Suddenly, three. Three seats for a movie. Three seats in a shoe store, or a waiting room, or a dentist's office.

And three seats at the Beaumont Hospital radiation clinic in Royal Oak, Michigan, on a Monday morning, where a nurse came out and asked if you were ready to get a "special helmet," and you shrugged and said "OK." We stood and walked together, all of us holding hands, one, two, three, down a long hallway and into the fray.

It is July of 2015 and sweltering hot, my first trip back to the mission since Chika left. She is the only one of our children to ever go to America, and I am not inside the gates thirty seconds before the other kids surround me and the questions start.

"Does Chika live with you?"

"Does Chika sleep in your house?"

"Does Chika have her own room?"

"Does Chika have a dog?"

They ask when Chika is coming back. They tell me they are saving her bed and no one else is sleeping in it.

The next day, I hang a drawing Chika made in the school office. It says, "Hi, everybody. I am playing and having fun. Love, Chika. P.S. I miss you."

The kids stare at it. She is different to them now, outside the gates, under my care. One of our girls asks if she can go to America, too, and I say no, not right now.

"But why?" she says. "I don't have a mother, either."

Us

———

"Mister Mitch?"

Hmm?

"Why did you keep this?"

Chika reaches between a stapler, coffee cups, rubber bands, and a tissue box (my desk looks like the sale bin at Office Depot) and holds up a picture frame: inside is a school questionnaire from Haiti that she filled out just two weeks before coming to the United States.

By "Name" she wrote "5." By "Age" she wrote "Chika."

At the bottom, she was asked to finish this sentence:

"When I grow up I want to be _____."

She wrote a single word.

BIG.

"Why did you keep it?" Chika repeats.

How do I answer? Because it once made us laugh? Because later it made us cry? Because I stare at it now and argue with God over why such a simple request could not have been granted?

When I grow up I want to be . . . BIG.

I don't know, Chika. Some things you just keep.

"I got big," she says.

When?

She drops her eyes.

"Don't you re-MEM-ber?" She fills her cheeks with air, like she's blowing up a balloon.

I push back in my chair.

I remember, I say.

———

Dexamethasone is a corticosteroid meant to reduce inflammation. Chika started taking it in advance of the radiation treatment, little pills she would swallow with applesauce. As a sports journalist, I had covered athletes who used steroids to bulk up, and when I first heard the doctors talk about this drug as "Dec," for its brand name, Decadron (*"How much Dec is she on?" "We could increase her Dec"*), it sounded almost sports-like. Ballplayers using steroids would call it "getting big." And indeed, in a short time, Chika got big, but not the way they did.

The steroids shrunk the tissue near the tumor but inflated her everywhere else. Her appetite grew ravenous. Her breakfast went from one banana to three eggs, cereal, grapes, and two pieces of toast with almond butter. At dinner, she could eat as much as I could. We were careful not to indulge these heightened cravings with junk food, but Chika's hunger was not discerning. She'd eat two helpings of salmon. Brussels sprouts. Caesar salad. If she saw me eating anything, her voice would skip up high. "Mister Mitch, what's thaaaaat?" I'd say, "It's a turkey sandwich." And she'd look away and mumble, "I wish *I* had a turkey sandwich."

In less than two months on steroids, Chika looked like someone else. She had a double chin, and her cheeks were so full, you'd have thought she was storing walnuts. I learned there is a medical term for this, *moon facies,* or moon face, something a mean kid might holler, and I worried about what other kids would say to Chika. Her arms and legs had dimpled, and her tummy protruded noticeably. She went from forty-eight pounds to seventy-three.

None of this diminished her joy. Her smile was just as bright, but instead of spreading across her face, it was puckered between her cheeks. Her mouth and eye still drooped down on the left, and she still walked with a hitch in her left leg, but the doctors said this might change if the radiation was effective.

I learned that despite the great complexity of the human brain, all an invader like DIPG had to do was to press against a certain spot on a certain lobe and boom—your eye drooped, your legs buckled, your speech drawled. Diminish the pressure, and the symptoms disappeared. It was almost too mechanistic, as if you could yell "Back off!" to the tumor and everything would return to the way it was.

The radiation was to serve that purpose, a beamline of subatomic particles, narrowly aimed and as destructive as a bomb. Every morning, five days a week, Chika would slide into a massive machine, her head locked down by a helmet, her eyes with little choice but to look up into the cylinder. The nurses who prepped her were endlessly upbeat—"You're amazing, Chika! You're a rock star!" Still, I wonder what the rock star thought when those nurses had to leave the room before the machine turned on.

All told, she did six weeks of this. We introduced routines to make it more fun—she signed herself in when she arrived, she picked out music to listen to during the session. But Chika's body paid a price. The hair behind her right ear disappeared, because radiation will destroy healthy cells along with cancerous ones, particularly fast-growing ones like hair cells. At night, sometimes, she would sweat and flop around the bed, yelling, in Creole, *"Doktè! Doktè!"*

Still, over time, there was significant shrinkage of the tumor, beyond what they had hoped. Her radiation oncologist, Dr. Peter Chen, showed us images on large computer screens and MRI scans. *You see this? That's when she first got here. Now look.* By early autumn, when I took her to a cider mill to feed the ducks and taste some apple pie, Chika's tumor had retracted by twenty-five percent.

Twenty-five percent?

"Maybe even thirty," Dr. Chen said.

We were filled with a sense of strength. With her initial at bat, Chika had smacked a solid triple. "She is going to beat this," Janine told me. "Why can't she be the first?"

As time passes, Chika acquires clothes, some that we buy her, some that our friends bring her. She likes to dress up, the frillier the better. She marches around in Janine's high heels. She drapes herself in multiple necklaces. She wears two hats at the same time.

"She likes to gild the lily," Janine jokes.

One day Chika and I are heading out.

"Hold on," I say. "You have something on your face."

"What?" she says.

I grab a napkin. I pat the area around her lips.

"You're kind of wet here. How did you get all wet?"

"Mister Mitch!" She throws up her hands. "That's my lip gloss!"

Us

―――

Summer is over before Chika appears again. I switch from shorts to long pants, and turn off the ceiling fans in the office. Chika always liked this office. When she came through the door she would lift her eyes to the tall bookshelves. She knew this was where I wrote, and that I needed quiet when I did. Perhaps getting to enter made her feel special.

This time, when she arrives, she taps me from behind and I nearly jump out of the chair. She laughs hysterically.

"What are you doing?" she asks.

Writing.

"About me?"

Like you wanted me to.

"Hmmph."

She spins to the piano behind us.

"Let's play something."

I have always had a piano in my office, owing to my earlier days as a musician. Even now, when I get lost in the woods of writing, I turn to playing to guide me out. Chika starts whacking the keys, making the same cacophony she made when she was alive.

"Don't bang," I used to scold. Then one day, I brought her to visit a friend, a jazz musician, who listened calmly as she pounded, then stood over her and created a bass line with his left hand and some chords with his right, a tuneful bed to envelop her wanderings. That was the last time I told Chika what to play. Everything in this world is music if you can hear it. Make a joyful noise, the psalm says.

We sit and tap out "Jingle Bells." Christmas songs were always welcome, even in summer. I sing, *Dashing through the snow, in a one-horse open sleigh, over fields we go—*

"Through the fields," she corrects.

Through the fields?

"Yeah."

Not "over" fields?

"No. See." She sings, *"Dashing through the snow, in a one-horse open sleigh, through the fields we go . . ."*

I start to sing with her, but she puts her hand over my mouth, then finishes with, *"laughing all the way, ha-ha-HΛ!"*

You have to do that? I ask, smiling.

She grins. Most times we sang, Chika cupped her palm over my mouth, a clear sign that her act was solo. It made me laugh then. It makes me laugh now.

"Mister Mitch? Why did you write those words?"

Which words?

She slides off the bench and moves to the desk. She points at the yellow pad, and number three on the list.

"Them," she says.

Lesson Three

———

A SENSE OF WONDER

We took you to Disneyland once, Chika. Do you remember? It was after the radiation treatments. You had been wondering about Sleeping Beauty's Castle, which they show at the start of every Disney movie. "Is that real?" you'd ask, and we'd say that it was, and someday we would take you to see it. One night, after putting you to bed, Miss Janine and I looked at the missing patch of hair above the back of your neck. Your forehead was perspiring. And we said to each other, "What are we waiting for?"

We made the reservations. We flew to California. I bought tickets for a weekday, hoping for smaller crowds, and we arrived before the park even opened.

What I remember most is what you did first. We entered through Main Street, passing souvenir shops. The rides were up ahead, and I wondered which would make you scream, "Can we do *that* one?"

Instead we passed a small pond, and a gray duck wandered

out of the water. And with Astro Orbitor to your right, Thunder Mountain to your left, and Sleeping Beauty's Castle straight ahead, you pointed down and yelled, "Look! A duck!" And you chased after it and giggled wildly, "Duck! Duck!"

I glanced at Miss Janine, who was smiling, too. With all those amusement park attractions calling, you got low to marvel at another living creature.

———

If the first words from a child's mouth are "Mommy" or "Daddy," the next word must be "Look!" That's how it felt to me, anyhow. As an uncle, I watched countless times as nieces and nephews held up scribblings—"Mommy, look!"—or prepared to pool dive—"Daddy, look!"—or grabbed a toy off a store shelf—"Uncle Mitch, look!" As dutiful family, we would nod and say, "Very nice" or "Wow."

But I confess a sense of disconnect. It was never as fascinating to me as it was to them.

Then you came along, Chika. And maybe because I'm older now, or maybe because your eyes were so much wider than mine, or maybe because it's simply different when the child is in your care, something stirred. I began to lean over, to see tiny miracles the way you saw them. Baby ducks running. Frogs hiding in the weeds. The wind lifting a leaf you were about to grab. One of the best things a child can do for an adult is to draw them down, closer to the ground, for clearer reception to the voices of the earth.

You did that for me, Chika. We buried in leaves. We studied ants in the driveway. We rolled in snow—which astonished you the first time you saw it—and made your very first snowman. You put me on the other end of a magnifying glass or a toy telescope, and through those lenses, I could marvel at the world the way you did. You were an unfailing antidote to adult preoccupation.

All you had to say was, "Look!"

Look. It's one of the shortest sentences in the English language. But we don't really look, Chika. Not as adults. We look over. We glance. We move on.

You looked. Your eyes flickered with curiosity. You caught fireflies and asked if they had batteries. You unearthed a penny and asked if it was "treasure." And without prompting, you knew discovery should be shared.

"*You* smell it," you would say, holding out a fragrant flower.

"*You* eat it," you would say, holding out a chocolate candy.

So I did. I followed your lead. I ran after you sledding. I rode behind your carousel horse. I splashed after you in the swimming pool, remember? You invented a game where one pool edge was America and one was Haiti and you paddled between them, bringing rice and beans back and forth, saying, "Here you go! Eat them! Yum!" I don't know where you came up with that, Chika, or why it made you cackle with laughter. But I swam beside you from country to country, and your imagination was a thing to behold.

Children wonder at the world. Parents wonder at their children's wonder. In so doing, we are all together young.

———

So you taught me that, Chika. Or rekindled it, if that sense of wonder remains a pilot light inside us all. There was such a timeless quality to your enterprises—crawling under tables on a secret mission, setting up tiny cups for an imaginary tea party—that it almost erased the urgency that hung over you.

But my receptors, being the grown-up kind, could not ignore that urgency.

The relative success of the radiation treatments had boosted our hopes, and even boosted your lips and left eye, closer to a normal symmetry. Your walking improved. You ran and danced. The summer passed and you were better than before. So, progress, right?

Still, I had been warned by doctors that this could be a "honeymoon" period, that the invader in your brain stem was "dormant" but not gone, a volcano regathering.

Be vigilant, I told myself. *Be wary.*

———

This was brought home to me during, of all things, a college football game in mid-September, at the massive University of Michigan stadium, which is affectionately called The Big House.

There were more than a hundred thousand people there that Saturday, and from my perch in the press box, where I had come to write my sports column, I glanced down just before the game began to see a family walking onto the field. The public-address announcer bellowed, *"Joining the captains for the coin toss is Chad Carr. Our thoughts and prayers are with the Carr family."*

I swallowed hard. The Carr family meant Lloyd Carr, the former Michigan football coach, whom I knew well, his son Jason, Jason's wife, Tammi, and their three children, including their youngest, Chad, who was four years old, and whom the announcer had individually recognized.

Because Chad Carr—like you, Chika—was suffering from DIPG.

I watched him carried out, listless in his father's arms, a beautiful child with a mop of blond hair. His battle had become a well-known story in Michigan, the subject of TV news reports and articles. I had spoken with Tammi several times. She told me all she knew about the disease, and introduced me to a community of families, all climbers on a worldwide DIPG mountain, sharing what ledge to grab, what slips to avoid, and sometimes, painfully, the news of those who had fallen. These families had a trust that strangers otherwise would not, phoning each other on nights and weekends. But with no historical path to defeat DIPG, they all, at some point, had to make a choice, without assurance it would work.

I dreaded that part of the conversation: *"So what do you think you'll do?"* It felt like those disaster movies, where one group decides to take the roof and the other takes the stairs, and you know they won't both make it out alive.

Our thoughts and prayers are with the Carr family. What did that mean? Had there been a setback? I knew his parents were trying everything. He was in his twelfth month since diagnosis. You, Chika, were in your fourth.

A honeymoon period. Dormant but not gone. The doctors' warnings never left my mind. I came home that day and you were eating with Miss Janine.

"Mister Mitch, we are having pink fish!" you yelled, meaning salmon. I pulled Miss Janine aside.

"Chika's having a good day," she said.

"I see that."

She looked in my eyes. "What's the matter?"

I hesitated.

"It might not last," I said. "We've got to keep pushing."

One night Janine is reading Chika a Veggie Tales book. It talks about believing in God.

"Does God have powers?" Chika asks.

"Yes," we say.

"Is He brave?"

"Yes."

"Does He protect horses?"

No idea where that came from.

"God protects everything," we respond.

"God created the whole, wide world," she says, singsongy, "and the uni-versity!"

"The universe?"

"Yeah, yeah, the universe. Whatever."

Me

I went to college with several guys who became doctors. I remember visiting one of them during the 1980s, when AIDS was rampant. I said something about how unbeatable the disease seemed.

"They'll find a cure for AIDS faster than they'll find one for cancer," my friend said.

That struck me. Years later, when Morrie Schwartz indoctrinated me to the world of ALS, I heard something similar. "They'll find a cure for ALS before they find one for cancer."

Cancer loomed like a dark cloud for as long as I can remember, impervious and imperious. I watched my uncle die from pancreatic cancer when he was forty-four—and I was twenty-one. My brother began a lifelong battle with cancer when he was just twenty-nine. Janine's sister Debbie fought a fifteen-year war with breast cancer, before finally, defiantly, succumbing. We buried her at fifty-six.

But a child? A grade IV brain tumor? This was not a fight I had prepared for. As a result, my education was fast and eye-opening. It often left me angry. I already knew the incredible profits in chemotherapy, and how those profits led to an insidious push for that treatment: when patients suggested another approach, physicians could be condescending, dismissing alternatives as risky, unproven, even quackery.

Janine and I were hardly physicians. But we knew this much: there was no evidence of chemo success with DIPG.

A new way up the mountain needed to be found.

———

"Did you know," a doctor named Mark Souweidane told me on a visit to Memorial Sloan Kettering hospital in New York, "that when we put chemo through an IV to treat a brain tumor, only three percent of it actually gets to the brain? There's something called a blood/brain barrier, a membrane that's very selective about what it lets in. Three percent. The rest just stays in the bloodstream."

This was a revelation to me—and a strong argument against conventional chemotherapy. Why shoot arrows to try and hit a pin?

Souweidane, a tall, thoughtful man with close-cropped hair, was determined to find a better way. He had grown up in Michigan with a penchant for fixing things. Early in his career, he started working on DIPG. He thought he'd have it licked "in two years."

Twenty-five years later, he was still crafting a battle plan. He'd begun a clinical trial of something called "convection enhanced delivery" (CED). Simply put, CED got much closer to the problem by placing a tube into the brain stem and slow-feeding cancer-killing drugs directly into the tumor.

The approach was risky. Putting anything directly into the brain always is. And as a trial, it meant all sorts of paperwork, agreeing to be studied, multiple trips back to Sloan Kettering for follow-ups. And no guarantees.

But here was a compassionate doctor focusing directly on DIPG, and Chika qualified for his program. If we were to really climb this mountain, if, as Janine said, "Why can't she be the first?," we would have to trek a new route.

We booked a hotel room.

We packed a bag.

We flew to New York City.

We are all in the car. I am driving. Janine and Chika sit in the back.

Chika starts singing.

"Doe, a deer, a email deer . . ."

"It's 'female,' sweetheart," Janine says.

Chika stops.

"What?"

"A 'female' deer. Not an 'email' deer. Female means 'a girl.' Those are the words."

Chika thinks for a moment. She crosses her arms.

"No!"

"No?"

"It's my mouth! I can say what I want!"

You

——

I want to write about your voice, Chika, because I think about it often, and I hear it all the time.

Every child has a feature that jumps out when you meet them. *The kid with the long curls. The kid with the weird laugh.* Yours was your voice. It reflected you perfectly. It was a chameleon, ever-changing. High-pitched and booming during the day. Lilting and tender at night. A sweet sandpaper in the mornings, so scratchy that Miss Janine and I would privately joke, "She hasn't been smoking, has she?"

It was a drawled-out "Yeaaaah" when you reluctantly agreed with us; it was a cannon shot "WHY?" when you didn't get your way. It was the whimper of a fairy when you said, "I'm sorry," and a peacock's squawk when you won a game. (I remember us playing tic-tac-toe and you cooing, "Bye-bye!" when you won. Trash talk from a five-year-old.)

Your voice was made for music, Chika, you had great pitch, and you often sang softly to yourself in the evenings; but when you wanted to, you could belt like Ethel Merman. One time, Miss Janine was helping you put on your night-gown, and as you wiggled through the sleeves, you were singing "L-O-V-E" by Nat King Cole, which they use in the movie *The Parent Trap*. When you got to the end, and sang that love was meant for me and "YOUUUUU," you spread your arms and threw back your head, as if a massive concert hall audience were wildly applauding. What joy you brought to your performance!

Your voice was a weather vane, it told us how your wind was blowing. When we flew to New York, you were particularly verbal: you asked me many questions, you were funny with the flight attendant, and you counted down from twenty until the wheels touched the tarmac. As we rose to deplane, a man who'd been sitting behind us said, "Excuse me, I just have to tell you, your daughter has the sweetest voice."

I was so touched by that. I made sure you thanked him for the compliment, never mentioning the effect the words "your daughter" had on me.

They say eyes are the reflection of the soul, Chika, but your voice was its echo, and we miss it every day. It was all the things you are, or were, or are still somewhere else, when you are not here with me in the mornings, rolling on the maroon carpet.

Us

———

"Mister Mitch?"

Yes?

"I didn't like New York so much."

You hated it. That's what you told me.

"I don't hate things now."

She flips onto her back.

Well, you liked it at the beginning.

"I liked the big toy store."

You sure did.

"But not the hospital."

Most people don't like hospitals.

"Why did you take me there?"

To New York?

"Uh-huh."

I push back in my chair. I think for a moment.

Hope, I say. Do you know what I mean? Hope? Is it a good reason to do something?

"Yeah," she sighs, rolling onto her belly. "It's a good reason."

———

By the time we flew to New York, Chika had become quite used to air travel. She handed her ticket to the TSA workers. She marched through the metal detectors in her light-up sneakers. She often needed to use the bathroom, and if we traveled without Janine, I would guide her to the airport ladies' rooms, then stand dutifully outside, looking at my watch.

One time she was taking particularly long. I began to worry. A middle-aged woman in a long coat saw me shifting on my feet and said, "Can I help you?" I explained the situation, and she kindly went inside and yelled, "Is there a Chika in here?"

A long pause.

"Who is calling me?"

I suppressed a smile.

"There's a man waiting outside for you," the woman said.

"I know, I know!" Chika hollered back. "That's Mister Mitch!"

When she emerged, she put her little hand in mine, her fingers moist from washing. "I had to poop," she said, and we walked on.

———

I realize in reading these words that it is easy, at times, given Chika's personality, to forget about her illness, and there were moments during that first year when we almost did. She was so often joking, dancing, her energy so boundless, that to the outside observer, no one would guess there was anything wrong. Even as her face and body changed, she marveled at herself in the mirror, and shook her newly substantial hips. Many kids would have at least asked why they were getting bigger. But Chika had such a bedrock of self-esteem. Nothing in a mirror seemed to shake it.

Still, certain words never left my mind. *The honeymoon period. Dormant but not gone.* It was what pushed us to New York in the first place. We didn't want to hold the tumor at bay; we wanted to eradicate it.

The night before Chika's CED procedure, Janine and I walked her around a jammed Times Square. She marveled at the multistory billboards and neon lights. Characters dressed as Spider-Man, Olaf, and Buzz Lightyear wandered freely through the crowds, and she ran up to them, wanting to talk. As we were leaving, one character removed his giant head and ran his hands through his sweaty hair. "Hey!" Chika squealed. "There's a man inside Mickey Mouse!"

Later, we went to the massive Toys "R" Us store, four stories high, with a small Ferris wheel inside. The three of us squeezed into a pink cart. Chika laughed when it started to move but hooked her arms around Janine's as it rose, making a frightened whimper.

We were feeling nerves of our own. Earlier in the day, I had again signed forms recognizing the risks of Chika's upcoming surgery. This time "paralysis" and "death" were among the potential outcomes. Dr. Souweidane, who was passionate about this trial and used the word *elegant* in describing the science of cancer research, signed them, too.

He then said he wanted to ask me something, and I said all right. He was fascinated by people's motivations, he explained, so could I tell him why I chose to do this? To bring Chika up from Haiti, pay all her medical expenses (at the start, without health insurance, most of Chika's treatments required us paying out of pocket) exploring all these various options, when she wasn't my child?

I was taken aback. I had never been asked "Why?" before. I think I answered that I never saw it as a choice. And whose child she was really didn't matter.

But then I had a question for him: Why is it that certain doctors, experts in the field, will advise you one way about battling cancer, while others equally expert will advise you another?

He crossed his legs and nodded, as if I'd just turned a tumbler in a lock. "The truth is, we don't know. Even in this trial, I don't know if this is the right agent that I'm using. Nobody does. But we can't just sit there like we have for decades, doing the same old thing."

That night in the hotel room, as we readied for bed, I found myself studying Chika, thinking the worst: What if something goes wrong? What if this is the last night we can speak to her? Dr. Souweidane was clear: one misplacement of the catheter, and the girl we knew could be gone.

"Mister Mitch, why are you looking at me?" Chika finally asked. I couldn't say the truth: that I was trying to memorize her. That I was thinking we'd been blessed with the best possible child under the worst possible circumstances.

Instead, I shrugged and mumbled, "Sorry."

She shook her head with her lips pursed, as if tasting those invisible lemons.

"It's OK," she decided. "You can look."

The next morning, Chika was wheeled into an operating room with the sun barely visible in the New York sky. Janine and I found chairs in the waiting area and passed the time with lukewarm coffee and half-eaten snacks. We read. We checked our watches. We got up and walked around. The CED process was like planning a space voyage. Hours were spent with computer models to set the catheter's path to the brain. Precision was critical. There was no hurrying.

Finally, in the early afternoon, Dr. Souweidane emerged, relieved to report that so far it had gone smoothly. We were able to see Chika, who was sleeping in a rolling bed, a large patch of her hair shaved off above her forehead. A tube was sticking out of her cranium, bolted in place. We were told it would stay in for up to twelve hours while an antibody with radioactive iodine was slowly dripped through it, directly into the tumor.

Given the potency of that agent, if we wanted to spend the night with Chika, they said, we would have to sleep behind a half wall lined with lead, to protect ourselves from radiation.

We also had to wear small devices to monitor our exposure. We were warned not to get too close to her, and never for more than a few seconds. It felt like we were in a nuclear plant and Chika had gone radioactive.

Although they encouraged us to sleep somewhere else, neither Janine nor I wanted to leave Chika on her own. She fights; we fight. So we slumped into the chairs behind the leaded walls and promised to tell each other if we started glowing. The night fell, and it lasted a long time.

Four

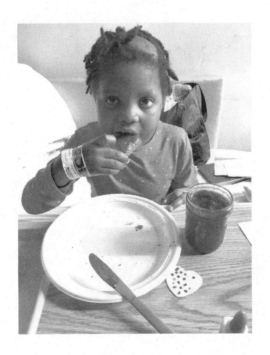

Bedtime at our orphanage is just after evening devotion. The children disperse and drag to their rooms. The youngest ones, weary from the day's heat, are often asleep in the arms of the nannies. The older ones wander in circles, using any excuse to stay outside. There is little else to do. No television. No computers. No phones. When the city power goes out, which it does every night, we dwell in complete darkness until someone revs up the generator.

I go from room to room and tell bedtime stories to each group, tales of princesses and unicorns for the younger children, tales of high schoolers with superpowers for the older ones. Afterward, I kiss each of them good night. Now and then, if the little girls ask for one, I will sing a song, and they grow quiet and attentive, an audience on their tummies. I read somewhere that the first music ever made might have been a lullaby. Anyhow, it helps them sleep.

When Chika came to America, I asked if she wanted a lullaby before lights-out. She said OK, so I sang her one, and I repeated it the next night and the next. It became our little routine, my sitting on her bed just before she nodded off, stroking her head while singing the melody to "Brahms' Lullaby." I made up these lyrics:

Lullaby and good night
Go to sleep now, little Chika
Lullaby and good night
Off to beddy-bye you go
Lullaby and good night
Go to sleep now, my darling
Lullaby and good night
Off to dreamland you go.

I doubted she was listening to the words. She would fall asleep, and that was good enough. But months later, Janine and I had to go out of town, and Chika stayed with friends of ours named Jeff and Patty. Late that night, I got a video message.

"Chika wanted to say something to you," Patty wrote.

In a darkened bedroom, Chika, in her nightgown, looked into the lens and began to sing:

"Lullaby and good night
Go to sleep now, my darling
Lullaby and good night
Go to sleep like we do!"

Then she added, "Good night, Mister Mitch!" and blew a kiss. To this day, I cry when I watch that.

Me

———

I should tell you where my notions of fatherhood come from, Chika.

My father was a good man. He lived to be eighty-eight. You met him once, when he was gray and stooped and confined to a wheelchair. But when he was younger, he looked a good deal like I do now, although his whiskers were thicker and he combed his hair back in the style of the day.

His name was Ira, and he grew up in Brooklyn, a middle child, like me, between a sister and a brother. His father, my grandfather, was a Polish immigrant, a plumber, who taught his son to work with his hands only until he could work with his mind. My father went from high school to college to the air force to an accountant job. He was not one to wander.

My grandfather was quiet, and my father would follow suit, and we, his children—my brother, sister, and me—grew up expecting the words that came from his mouth to matter. I can never recall the man going on about anything. He said what he had to say and was done with it. He had a deep, baritone voice (he once dreamed of being an opera singer), which made even his simple remarks sound serious. He was serious most of the time.

My father was an early riser, fond of coffee and big band music and reading the newspaper, a patient, industrious, and impeccably groomed man. His suits were always pressed and his shirts were always tucked in, even on weekends. He made us scrambled eggs with salami, which we loved, and albacore tuna salad, which he mashed so diligently, it was as spreadable as butter. He never sought attention. He had no hobbies that took him away from us. No golf. No card games. He embraced the value system passed down to him, that a man provides for his family and his contentment is found in that.

But there was, beneath his efficiencies, a warm, protective aura, a soul upon whom others could rely. When my mother's father died of a heart attack—she was sixteen at the time—it was my father, only seventeen, who stepped in and took control of the household. Although they'd been dating less than a year, he cooked breakfast for my mother's family, did chores in the afternoons, and became a dad to her young brother. That's a lot of responsibility for someone still in high school, but if you knew my father, you would say it suited him. He was, from my earliest memories, the person others came to, for advice, or aid, or money. He did not flinch from these requests, but as the years passed I wondered if he ever missed not having a carefree, youthful stage. Sometimes life throws a saddle on you before you are ready to run. In any case, he never complained.

Finding Chika

I always felt safe around my father. I have a memory of swimming with him in a local lake when I was maybe six years old. We would go there on hot summer days, many families did, and I was paddling away to explore, the way children do.

"Don't go too far now," my father said, but I kept going until it felt like I'd reached foreign waters. Suddenly, some older boys who were horsing around pointed at me and yelled, "Let's get him!" I don't know what motivated them, or how serious they were, but I remember feeling terrified, acutely aware of the distance I had drifted from my dad. I swam as I had never swum before, splashing wildly, gulping water, certain those older boys were going to grab my legs and pull me to some hidden underwater prison. As I reached my father, I hurled my arms around his midsection, gasping for air. When I peeked out, the boys had gone.

My dad barely moved. He never asked what happened. But to this day, I can still feel his waist in my wet grip, and the comfort it gave me. For many years, that was my perception of fatherhood, a place where a child can find sanctuary. Perhaps this is why I took over the orphanage. Perhaps I've grown into my father that way.

As I said, you met him once, Chika, when we took a trip to his small, one-story home in California. Remember? This was less than a year after my mother died, and he was diminished by her death more than I can explain, even beyond the strokes that robbed him of walking and clear speech. They had been married sixty-four years; he was heartbroken without her. I'd hoped that meeting you might lift his spirits.

When we arrived, I said, "Chika, this is my daddy," and you were hesitant, perhaps surprised that I had one. But you hugged him and called him "Pop Pop." He noticed your flowered headband and said, weakly, "That's very pretty."

Later, you sat on a couch across the room and joked with his nurses. You were being silly and noisy and he turned to me and said, "She's very loud, no?" I tried to remind him of your backstory, your medical challenges, all the treatments we were trying. I'd shared this many times with him over the phone, but I never knew what he remembered. In the old days, my father always responded thoughtfully. Near the end, he mostly shrugged. Age is such a thief.

As we watched you joking around, I mentioned that you'd been here six months already.

"I had no idea how much effort this took," I said.

He coughed and straightened in his wheelchair. I wasn't sure he'd heard me. Then, in a thin voice, he said, "That's what having kids is."

When my father died, Chika, I felt rudderless in this world, with a deep, anguished yearning for a comfort no longer there. I missed him more than I even imagined I would, and my brother and sister told me the same thing. He was a man more appreciated once he was gone, no longer doing all those things you took for granted.

They say as you age you become more and more like your

parents. And perhaps that is true. If so, if I ever offered you security the way my dad offered it to me, then I am glad. I know I tried. I remember times when you and I were walking and, without prompting, you reached out and took my hand, your little fingers sliding into mine. I would like to tell you how that felt, but it is too big for words.

I can only say that it made me feel like a father, and nearly all of what I learned about that role, I learned from the man who raised me, and the rest I learned from you. Perhaps it is no coincidence that the day we buried him was the day you came back to me. I think about that a lot.

———

By the way, I mentioned those headbands. You had many of them. Pastels, polka dots, each with a large flower clip, which we positioned over the left side of your forehead to cover the bald spot where the doctors had shaved you. You discovered that bald spot quite accidentally, the day after your CED procedure at Sloan Kettering.

Dr. Souweidane told us things had gone well. The radioactive agent had distributed widely into the tumor. Now we just had to wait for its effect. Miss Janine and I were collapsed in the hospital chairs. You needed to use the bathroom. Miss Janine rose slowly and guided you in, still half-asleep.

Suddenly, I heard a scream.

"HEY! What happened to my HAIR?"

We'd forgotten about the mirror.

"HEY!" you kept yelling, "HEY, GUYS!"

You weren't angry as much as bemused. You rubbed your scalp and said it felt funny. We gave you a wool cap and you liked that just fine and you wore it with your hospital pajamas until we found those flowered headbands, which you liked even more. For the next few months, that was your look whenever we went out. You wore one, two, or three flowers on that headband, along with frilly tops, colorful tights, a furry coat, and flashing shoes. No one even knew about the bald patch. Such a dazzling little package you were.

Us

———

It is two months before I see Chika again. I sort through photographs. I watch videos. But the mornings come and go and there are no visits, just digital reminders of her face and voice.

As I write more pages, I consider the obvious: that her appearances are purely my imagination. But if that is true, why can't I summon her at will? When I try, it's as fruitless as summoning a dream.

October passes. November nears an end. Thanksgiving arrives, a three-day tradition in our family, and on Thursday morning, several of my cousins knock on the front door early, ready to begin preparing the food. Still in my bedclothes, I let them in, then head down to my office for the last moments of privacy before our house is packed.

I put away some papers. I close down the computer.

"Where are you going, Mister Mitch?"

Chika is leaning against the bookcase, in a long pink sleeping shirt, blue tights, and rabbit slippers. Her knees are pulled up and wrapped by her arms.

Good morning, beautiful girl.

"Where are you going?"

No good morning?

"Good morning, Mister Mitch."

I was going upstairs.

"Why?"

Because there are people up there. And more coming. It's Thanksgiving.

"When you eat orange potatoes?"

Sweet potatoes. Yes.

She thinks for a moment.

"We can hide."

From the family?

"Yeah."

But I like them.

"You can hide from people you like."

Why would you do that?

"So they can find you!" Her little mouth falls open and her eyes go wide in disbelief. "Don't you want people to *FIND YOU*?"

I laugh, because her tone is so familiar. When she was alive, Chika was often aghast if you didn't follow her logic. I remember one morning when she sat at my desk, drawing doodles and singing "Supercalifragilisticexpialidocious." Suddenly, she stopped and banged the paper.

"Now *you* sing it," she insisted.

Me?

"Yeah. You sing it."

How do the words go?

She exhaled hard, then made the same face she's making now, pure childish exasperation. "You don't watch *MARY POPPINS* BEFORE?" she screamed. "Are you CRAZY?"

Sorry, I said, hiding a laugh.

"You just have to watch it again," she mumbled, returning to her drawing. "No problem."

That wasn't anger, by the way, more like experiencing life at such full intensity, she couldn't help but holler. At moments like those, I felt as if I were hanging onto Chika's magic carpet, with no idea where her mind was flying.

"You can hide with me here," she says now, pulling her knees closer. "We could get under a blanket."

Then what?

"Then they come look for you. And when they say, 'Where is Mister Mitch?' you jump out and say, 'Here I am!' And they say, 'Oh. Look. It's him!'"

Will they see you, too?

She smacks her lips. "No, no, no. They don't see me."

How come?

She doesn't answer.

Instead she says, "I'm going to Haiti." She pulls a blanket from the couch, drapes it over her head, and vanishes.

After six months in America, we take Chika home for Christmas. The holiday is a big deal at the mission, laden with traditions: a Nativity play; stockings hung in the dormitory; a once-a-year meal of goat, fried plantains and pikliz, a spicy pickled cabbage dish.

She is giddy with excitement. The night before, she crawls on the bed and tickles me until I beg her to stop. Then she asks what's going to happen, step by step.

As I go through it, her eyes drift away. She doesn't look like she did when she left Haiti. She's lost hair. She's lost teeth. The operations. The steroids. I ask if she is scared to be going back.

"A little scared," she says, making a small space between two fingers. "I'm crying happy tears."

She has never used that phrase before. Happy tears. I wonder where she gets such insight.

The next morning, for the big day, she wears white tights and sneakers, with a lime-green hoodie over a sleeveless top. We board the plane and she glues to the window. Many of the passengers are Haitian, and she occasionally spins and says, "Hey. They are talking like me!"

As soon as we land in Port-au-Prince, she runs up the jetway, *all but leaving me behind. The airport band starts playing, banjo, accordion, guitar, bongo drums, and she dances in the hallway, shaking and twirling in a way that proves she is home, because only home could liberate such joy.*

Alain meets us in baggage claim. We load in his vehicle, and Chika hides behind his seat as we drive through the mission gates. The kids have been informed of her return and they are chanting "Chika! Chika!" as we pull in. Alain looks back in amazement and says, "Do you hear this?"

"Don't look at me, Mister Alain!" she squeals. "Look at something else!"

When the car door opens, there is a massive rush and the nannies are shouting and the little kids are jumping and there are so many hands around her, lifting her up, as her face is smacked with kisses. When they finally put her down, she wiggles her little black shoes in the dirt. Then she pulls off the hoodie and runs to the swing set, jumps on a swing, and pushes herself higher, as the other kids gather and watch. If I could freeze any moment and give it to her as a gift, it might be this one, flying over the happy expressions of her brothers and sisters as they marvel at her return. I rub my eyes. Happy tears.

You

———

There's a support beam in our kitchen that runs floor to ceiling. At some point we decided to make it the family growth chart. We measured our nieces' and nephews' heights on their birthdays, then scribbled the year in pencil.

When you first arrived, Chika, we lined you up, too, and drew a mark where the top of your head met the plaster. We let you write CHIKA. And every few months, you wanted a new measurement. Your pencil marks remain to this day.

A child is like a little ball of time unfurling. But your time advanced on two levels, for as you grew, your Invader could grow, too, which made the passing months our friend and our enemy. You got taller. Your hair filled out. You lost baby teeth and collected monies from the Tooth Fairy. You learned capital letters and small letters. Your English improved greatly. If I spoke to you in Creole, you would roll your eyes and say, "Mister Mitch, we are in America now."

But there were also regular visits to hospitals, and blood tests, and constant MRIs of your brain, so frequent that one time, I was reminding you about lying still inside the machine, and you moaned and said, "I know, I know," and made your entire body rigid, just to prove it.

Our hope was to get through one month then the next, like swinging from vines through the medical jungle. Despite the dire predictions with DIPG—*nobody survives it*—there was always the chance something radical might be developed, some new laser treatment or stumbled-upon medication. A doctor at Stanford was having early success with a chemo drug called Panobinostat. There was talk of a progressive clinic in Mexico. A London-based group was doing multiport CED deliveries, much like Dr. Souweidane at Sloan Kettering, only with four catheters at a time.

Every night that you said your prayers, we later said our own, silently asking for someone in a lab, maybe halfway around the world, to be peering through a microscope and whispering, *"Look, it's working."* You reach for fantasies like that, Chika, when you need a weapon to beat the unbeatable. Your tumor had been operated on in June, diminished by radiation in July and August, and unaffected by other treatments from September to the following March.

That was good news and bad. No matter what we tried, including the CED process—which we actually repeated a few months later in New York—the tumor held its ground, a bear in a cave, not growling, but not going anywhere, either. The treatment Dr. Souweidane had put directly into your brain stem—which glowed green on a computer screen, verifying its excellent distribution—nonetheless had no real effect. I remembered my conversation with him (*"We don't know if this is the right agent"*) and fought the haunting sense that, despite their white coats and laboratories, these doctors, against this disease, were flying in the dark.

———

So meanwhile, Chika, we focused on making good memories. In January, after the Haiti visit, we organized your sixth birthday party, at a loud, animal-themed restaurant called The Rainforest Cafe. You were surrounded by kids—nieces, nephews, our friends' children—and you ran around the tables wearing a headpiece of stitched candles. We cheered when the cake came out, and Miss Janine and I held hands and whispered, "Eight months," remembering Dr. Garton's dire prediction that you might not live beyond four.

In February, I took you sledding for the first time. You cringed and shut your eyes at the top of the hill, but you shrieked in delight all the way down. When I caught up, your cheeks were wet from sprayed snow and you were laughing so hard you could barely get out the words: "Can we do it *again?*"

In March, we arranged for swimming lessons, because swimming was something you adored. You wore a bathing cap and goggles and looked like a pint-size aviator from the 1920s. You squealed when you splashed in and squealed when you resurfaced and you yelled, "Miss Janine! You come in! *You* come in!"

And then one day in April, having left you at your lesson, I drove to work. Ten minutes later, my cell phone rang. It was Miss Janine, but her voice sounded different, it was hurried and panicky.

"Come home right now. Chika just threw up in the pool."

"Malè pa gen klakson."

[Misfortune doesn't have a horn.]

—HAITIAN PROVERB

Lesson Four

———

KID TOUGH

Chad Carr passed away.

The cherubic little blond-haired boy whose father carried him onto the Michigan football field died exactly fourteen months after his DIPG diagnosis. I shivered when I heard the news. Janine started crying.

Because his grandfather was a famous coach, Chad's death made news across the country, and brought a rare spotlight to this horrific disease. People were reminded that Neil Armstrong, before he ever walked on the moon, lost his two-year-old daughter to the same affliction in 1962. Little had changed in all those years. DIPG remained a wrathful thief, preying on children, robbing families of their present *and* their future.

The Carr family started a foundation in their son's memory. They called it Chad Tough. And while you are not here for me to read this to you, Chika, I want to say what I have learned about that word, *tough*, because children, especially sick children, have a toughness unique to their young souls, one that can comfort even the fretting adults around them.

This is something you taught me.

This is fourth on my list.

Let me share an example. There was a night in Sloan Kettering hospital, during our second try at the CED process, when you were again being infused with the radioactive iodine antibody. It traveled from a large box, through a long tube, and down the catheter into your head.

This was around 3:00 a.m. I was sleeping in a chair across from your bed behind the leaded half wall. For some reason, my eyes flicked open, and in the darkness, I saw you standing right in front of me, your head tilted, like something from a horror movie. The catheter was poking up from your cranium, its cord stretched back as taut as a tightrope.

"Chika!" I screamed.

"I want to go to the toy store," you rasped.

I rushed you back to the bed, praying you hadn't yanked the catheter loose. I yelled for the nurses, who raced in, stunned. For the next hour, we waited anxiously until Dr. Souweidane arrived. He, too, was astonished. None of his patients had ever gotten out of bed during that procedure, let alone walk across a room.

Thankfully, you did no damage, and we all collapsed with relief. Come morning, you barely remembered it.

Kid Tough. I have been to many children's hospitals, and every visit pays witness to the word *resilience*: youths playing board games during chemo infusions, or holding IV poles as they hurry down hallways to an arts and crafts room.

You had that resilience, Chika. You had it in hospitals. You had it at the orphanage. In truth, you had it from your first week on Earth, when you slept in the fields with your mother and sisters. Even at the mission, when nearly all our kids contracted a painful, mosquito-spread virus called chikungunya, you simply lay in the gazebo with a cold towel on your head, enduring the symptoms.

That day you threw up in the pool, I rushed home to find Miss Janine holding you. You were wrapped in a towel, your eyes were lowered, and you smelled of chlorine. Still, you did not complain. You were mostly upset that you couldn't keep swimming.

We made a fast appointment at Mott's, where you had undergone your initial surgery. A small team there was following your case, two doctors in particular: a pediatric neuro-oncologist named Patricia Robertson (you called her "Dr. Pat") and a star researcher named Carl Koschmann ("Dr. Carl"), who, if he removed his white coat and pulled on a T-shirt, could easily have been imagined in the front row of a rock concert.

They made an interesting pair, at least thirty years apart in experience. You would walk for them, talk for them, have your reflexes and eyes examined by them. You got so used to this, you yawned your way through it. But they were measuring you on their own kind of growth chart, Chika, different from the pencil-marked beam in our kitchen.

Shortly after that pool incident, and eleven months after your original Haitian MRI, they told us the news we hoped we'd never hear:

The Invader had stirred.

The latest scans showed the tumor was growing. The small changes we had noticed—your left eye being less responsive, your gait being off—were related to this. The imbalance and pressure may have led to your vomiting.

Dr. Pat recommended we rev up the drug treatment. We debated the idea. Drugs against this foe still mostly meant chemotherapy. And chemotherapy hadn't cured anyone of DIPG. We called everyone we knew, seeking alternatives. But time was passing, and you were getting worse.

So, as much as we hated it, we slid you into the world of medications, because we had to keep fighting, to keep swinging for that next vine. Miss Janine read voraciously on brain disorders and consulted with cancer health experts, so in addition to the drugs the doctors prescribed, she added vitamins and supplements and probiotics to keep you strong. She gave you a giant "shake" of supplements every day—chocolate, vanilla, or strawberry flavored—which you started out liking and soon had to be coaxed into drinking.

Thankfully, you had no problem swallowing pills. You often made a game of it. Once in the back of a car, I placed a single pill on a spoonful of applesauce, and you bragged, "I can do two." I said, "Really?" and you said, "Watch. Watch!"

And you placed two pills in the applesauce, gulped the spoon, then stuck out your tongue.

"No way!" I said.

"No way . . . ," you repeated, happily, "José!"

You never asked what the pills were for. Instead you kept searching for laughs, as you did even in the unlikeliest moments. As your walking worsened, you'd sometimes stumble. But you'd grin and shout, "I fell on my BUTT!" When your foot began to tingle, a neurological consequence, you'd stomp it and say, "My foot is tickling me." As your eye and mouth drooped, you stared in the mirror and made funny faces, as if to challenge your new expression.

Watching your struggle was so difficult, Chika, and knowing what to say became equally hard. One day I saw you walk unsteadily to a shelf of toys. You grabbed a doll and fell backward. Then, as if deciding that walking wasn't worth it, you crawled with that doll tucked into your chest, until you reached a space beneath the kitchen island where you set up shop, bringing the world down to ground level.

I teared up, Chika, and I turned away so you wouldn't see me. As you played on the floor, accepting the new rules, your toughness far exceeded mine, and gave us comfort, even as we were trying to comfort you.

Us

———

"Mister Mitch?"

Hmm?

"Christmas is coming."

She sits in her little chair, wearing a blue dress, slippers, and a pink earflap hat. She pulls the flap cords down around her cheeks. She has appeared several times since vanishing on Thanksgiving morning, but her visits are shorter now, and she wears different clothes each time.

Do you remember all your Christmases? I ask.

"How many did I have?"

Well, you had two with your mommy.

"But I was so LITTLE!"

And one with your Godmommy.

"How many at the mission?"

Three.

"How many at your house?"

One.

"When?"

The last year.

She lets go of the earflaps.

"I know, I know." She sighs.

What?

"That's not a lot of Christmases for a little girl."

I didn't say that.

She taps her head. "You said it *here*."

You

One day I came home to find you playing a card game with our friend Nicole. You drew a card and she drew a card, and she made a joke and you laughed. It seemed perfectly normal, except Nicole was thirty-eight years older than you.

And she was on the younger end of your American playmates.

You went camping with our friends Jeff and Patty, who were already grandparents. Miss Janine's sisters Kathy and Tricia, in their fifties, would take you to get your nails painted. Our friend Dr. Val, in her sixties, would take you home to play with her dog.

You had a network of companions who ranged from two to five decades older than you, and while they were mostly our work colleagues or familial connections, you called them "my friends." You had a remarkable skill for collecting anyone you met; they would always ask to see you again. There was Margareth, a Haitian-born case manager; and Lyn and Carmella, both masseuses; and Anne-Marie, our sister-in-law; and Frank, Mark, Marc, and Jordan, who worked with me. Yoga teachers, deli owners, musicians, nurses. You were a pied piper of grown-ups, many of whose children were out of the house and who found in you a brief reconnection with the wonder of little souls.

Of course, you would have preferred some little souls of your own. And had Miss Janine and I been of normal parenting age, our nieces and nephews would have been your mates. But they were grown now, too. We tried taking you to places with other children—fairs, church events, holiday celebrations at a local heath cub. But sometimes other kids didn't know what to make of you and your challenges, and you'd walk back to us and say, "They didn't want to play with me."

You tried so hard. You jumped in line at a Halloween dance. You presented tea sets to other girls. But with new kids, you would get tongue-tied, you, of all people, and just hold out whatever you had, and they would sometimes take it and walk away. I studied your vacant look, hoping they would come back. It broke my heart.

You missed going to school. We tried to re-create that, but, given the constant medical attention, we could only homeschool you with lessons sent by my sister, Miss Cara, who runs our school at the orphanage, and friends like Miss Diane, a retired teacher who sat with you for hours doing spelling and mathematics. We even dressed you in your Haitian school clothes, a purple shirt, navy blue skirt, white socks and black shoes, so it would feel more like the mission.

But it wasn't the mission. The mission would have meant dozens of children, laughing and yelling and racing to their classrooms, not a lonely kitchen table overlooking our backyard.

———

Of course there *were* a few children you befriended in America. One of them was our nephew Aidan, who was eight when you arrived, and who took to you immediately. A soft-spoken, gently mannered boy, with thick, cowlicked brown hair, he played anything you wanted to play, and watched whatever you wanted to watch. And it was pretty clear, after several months, that you were, as my grandmother used to say, "sweet on him." You dressed up when he was coming over. You got bashful when he arrived. You were quieter, even deferential.

One time I took the two of you to an arcade near our house, and I changed a ten-dollar bill into quarters and put the quarters into Dixie cups. Had it just been you and me, you might have jokingly tried to take my cup. Instead, you looked at Aidan and said, "I have too much," and poured half your cup into his.

You and Aidan went on boat rides together and to the aquarium together, and one time at his house you danced together to a video of the Cha Cha Slide, and when he fell down you slapped him on the butt.

When you spoke about growing up and getting married, which you did all the time, we would tease you and men-tion Aidan's name and you would get a silly grin or say, "I dunno . . ." or "Maybe . . ."

And then one summer night, more than a year after you'd been with us, when your walking had deteriorated and your left eye no longer blinked and your therapies included sitting for hours with a needle in your arm, you were lying in bed, having just watched a princess movie. And you asked if you could one day marry a prince.

Miss Janine said, "What about Aidan? He's not a prince, but he's a really nice boy. Would you want to marry him?"

You made a face. "Aidan will not marry a girl like me."

We looked at each other.

"Why do you say that, Chika?"

"Because Aidan will not marry a girl who cannot walk."

You said it so innocently, so matter-of-factly, that it robbed us of our breath. And while we recovered to offer the standard adult response, that love doesn't care about sickness or health, inside we were trembling, because we saw in you something, with your disease, that we were terrified of seeing in ourselves.

Acceptance.

Although Chika is brave about almost every medical development, she is still scared of needles. She calls them "stickies." She can handle MRIs, radiation, even a catheter to her brain. But her eyes travel to a needle no matter how a nurse tries to hide it, no matter which way I cradle her head, and say, "Gade mwen, Chika," look at me. It's as if she can't help but watch.

To make things worse, she is a difficult blood draw. Her veins hide. "A tough stick" the nurses call her. This means the thing she hates the most, they have to keep repeating.

Chika has started on Avastin, a tumor-starving drug. To infuse it, she needs an IV in her arm. This is always difficult. But by June of 2016, more than a year into her diagnosis, it has grown impossible. They cannot get a vein.

On one particular visit, they try twice on her left arm, wrapping the mustard colored tourniquet around her biceps, rubbing the alcohol swab, sticking her. No luck. She is screaming. They switch to her right arm, wrap the tourniquet, find a spot, swipe the alcohol, stick her again.

"Nope," a nurse mumbles.

They bring in a vein specialist. She wraps a warm compress around Chika's hand. She taps the skin. Doesn't find a spot. She goes to the other hand. Repeats the process. "We can't do more than four tries," she notes.

She finally inserts a needle an inch from Chika's wrist. Chika howls.

"Make them stop!" she cries out.

"They're almost done, sweetheart, almost done."

"Make them stop, Mister Mitch!"

My heart is racing. I'm imploring them to finish. The IV finally takes. But seconds later, there is blood in the tube. The specialist frowns.

"What?" I say.

"We blew the vein."

They gather up their tools and force tight smiles as they leave. That's it. No infusion today. A nurse fetches someone to talk to me about putting a port under Chika's skin, inside her chest, because, she says, "This situation isn't going to get any better."

They offer Chika a cartoon sticker. She ignores it. I bundle her limp frame in my arms. Her cheeks are stained by tears. She gives me her hand, wet from wiping her nose, and whimpers something she never said before.

"I wanna go back to Haiti."

Me

———

Few things made Chika happier than eating. She tried almost everything. I remember a group of us sitting outside on a warm summer night, feasting on Lebanese food, and Chika singing, "Baba . . . ghan-*oush!*"—the word fascinated her—then laughing and eating more of it, then repeating, "Baba . . . ghan-*oush!*"

She was six.

Janine was adamant about her eating foods that helped her and avoiding those that might hurt. This included sugar, because of how it feeds cancer. Same for processed foods like chips and snacks.

But Chika was still a kid. She still longed for such things. Once, at a family party, I sat down on the couch and she slid a pillow between us.

"Are you trying to block me?" I asked, smiling.

"I don't want you to be mad," she mumbled.

"Chika, why would I be mad?"

She slowly moved the pillow.

She was hiding a bag of Cheetos.

Another time, she rode home from a wedding shower

with our friend Nicole. When Nicole checked the rearview, Chika was sound asleep. Only when they reached the house did Nicole discover Hershey's Kisses wrappers all over the seat. Chika had opened a gift basket and eaten all that chocolate at once.

Later, when Janine tried to tell me this story, Chika slapped her hands over my ears.

"No, no, no, no, no," she protested.

"What, Chika? Let me hear."

"OK. But don't freak out."

Freak out?

Of course, we were never mad over such things. On the contrary, we hated taking anything away from her. We hated doing anything that reminded her of her sickness. Janine cried when they told us we had no choice but to put that port inside Chika's chest, mostly because Chika would now have to see a plastic bump in her skin every day.

"Those things get infected," Janine said.

"What else can we do?"

"I don't trust it."

"You don't trust it." I sighed. "What's our alternative?"

The day after nurses used that port for the first time, I took Chika back to Haiti for my monthly visit. A reward for her perseverance.

It was mid-July, the hottest time of the year. Janine dressed her in white shorts and a lime-green T-shirt and a white headband with a big green flower on it. Chika wanted to arrive after the kids were sleeping and sneak into her bunk bed, so when the girls woke in the morning, they would all say, "Hey, look! It's Chika!" She reviewed this plan with military precision during our plane ride down.

She seemed particularly excited about this trip. Perhaps she was growing weary of America, the hospitals, the treatments. She could only walk on her own now with difficulty, and her left eye didn't close all the way, even when sleeping. Her hair was missing on the back side of her neck, and her thighs showed stretch marks from the severe weight gains and losses. Her mouth drooped into the shape of a sideways teardrop.

We also noticed her becoming less patient. More defiant. She often yelled "NO!" She hid under the table. There were consequences to such actions, because we refused to allow pity to replace teaching, and we wanted to teach her for the rest of a long life.

Once, when she refused to drink her supplement shake, Janine said, "Chika, we're just trying to take care of you." And she spun and yelled, "You're not here to take care of me! You're here for punishment and taking things away!"

I tried to intervene.

"Chika, if you want to go to Aidan's, you have to finish your shake."

"If you want to stay HERE, you have to finish YOUR shake!" she retorted.

I can't say these arguments didn't affect us. They hurt

sometimes. But we knew she was justified. Chika didn't rail against going to bed or finishing her vegetables. If she didn't want a medicinal milk shake, or to go for an MRI, could we blame her? We were always up against an invisible wall, not wanting to explain too deeply, not wanting to scare her or make her burden heavier.

We also never knew the extent of her pain; she dealt with so much, and so rarely complained. Sometimes she would say, "Mister Mitch, my head hurts," and while I would say "Let me rub it" or give her a children's aspirin, it would privately terrify me, because what if it wasn't just a passing headache?

In a way, I was sort of relieved when Chika argued with us, when she showed us her fight, as I knew she would need fight to get through this. So, OK, I figured. Argue if need be. Yell and scream. Do not go gently.

We arrived in Haiti late, and the kids were asleep by the time Alain's car pulled through the gates. Chika didn't look well; she was tired and sweating. I suggested she stay in my room until morning.

She didn't protest. I got her changed, and we said our prayers and she lay down on a small mattress. A few minutes later, she asked to sleep in my bed.

I lifted her head. I said, "Chika, what's wrong—"

And she vomited all over me.

My chin, my shoulders, and my shirt were covered. I

rushed her to the toilet, but she had already spit up everything. She was crying and I was saying "It's OK, it's OK," and she was sweating through her nightshirt, but she moaned that she was cold. I cleaned her up and placed a wet towel on her forehead, and I gave her some Tylenol to fight the fever. She fell into a troubled sleep, matched by my own.

Us

———

Two days before Christmas, Chika visits again.

"Look, Mister Mitch!"

I spin from my desk to see her standing in the doorway, wearing a yellow gown with layered skirts, a satin bodice, and ruffled sleeves. I remember buying her this outfit in New York, after her treatments at Sloan Kettering had finished. We'd taken her to the Disney Store to pick out one thing she wanted. She ran her hand over dolls and water bottles, but she stopped at the clothing.

"It's Belle's dress!" she marveled. *"Beauty and the Beast!"*

I lifted the hanger.

"Can I get it, Mister Mitch? *Please?*"

As if I could say no.

We have a photo of Chika in that dress and its matching tiara. She is standing in front of a full-length mirror, looking proudly at her reflection. I love that shot. It's the only picture we have of Chika smiling at herself.

Are you going out somewhere? I joke now.

"Where will I go?" she asks.

Nowhere. It's just something people say when they see someone dressed up.

"Mister Mitch?"

Hmm?

"Do you really see me?"

Yes. Why?

"Do you see me now?"

She is suddenly in the corner.

I still see you, I say.

"Are you sure?"

Yes.

She pulls at something on her gown.

"This dress is pretty."

Do you remember *Beauty and the Beast*, I ask?

"Yeah. It's about a girl who has to save her father."

I am about to correct her. But that's actually true.

Chika? I say. Why did you ask if I could see you?

She suddenly has a wand in her hand.

"I didn't," she whispers. "You did."

She waves the wand.

"Bibbidi-bobbidi-boo!" she yells, and disappears.

Chika's father is alive.

He is living in Tabarre, a forty-minute ride from the mission. At one point, we were told he was dead. Now we are told differently. Chika's godmother says she knows how to find him.

This is not uncommon in the Haitian orphan world. Adults who bring us children will sometimes say the parents are deceased to increase their odds of acceptance. Now and then, the parents will actually send someone in with their child and instruct them to lie. Although we try to verify everything, there are no digital records, no agencies that keep track of such things. You ask questions. You ask for documents. At some point, you accept what you are told or you do not.

On the trip that begins with Chika vomiting, I ask Alain to drive me to the father's house. We meander through traffic out to a rural, agricultural landscape. We park on a dirt road. We push through a wooden gate. There's a small square of land, with a large breadfruit tree. This is where Chika was born.

And stepping out in front of me is her father, Fedner Jeune.

He is small and compact, maybe five foot six, with a wide mustache, a full head of hair, and deep bags under his eyes, which are bloodshot red. They rarely meet mine.

*Alain handles the introductions and we speak, through transla-
tion. I ask about Fedner's upbringing. I ask about Chika's infancy.
He answers every inquiry with very few words.*

*He says he was there when Chika was born, but was not at
home when the earthquake happened. He says that for months, he
and Chika's mother lived apart, while he rebuilt the cinder block
house. He confirms that after she died, all four of his kids went to
live with other people. He doesn't say why.*

*The house, which has no door, is one room now, with a single
lightbulb for illumination. The ground nearby is spotted with bean
and banana plants. Water is drawn from a pump. There is no
bathroom; they use a latrine on a neighbor's property.*

*A woman and a little child sit playing beneath a tree. Alain asks
Fedner if this woman is with him, and he says, "Yes."*

Is this where Chika played? I ask.

"There," he says, pointing.

Is that the field she slept in after the earthquake?

"There." He points again.

*I ask if he knew Chika was being brought to us when she was
three.*

"Yes, I knew."

Did her godmother ask you or tell you?

"She told me."

And it was all right with you?

"It was all right with me."

*I don't ask why he didn't want Chika back, even though part of
me screams for an answer. I remind myself I can never know the
circumstances of his life, or its hardships. I remind myself he lost*

his partner, the mother of his children. Who knows how his world was overturned?

Instead, I explain the reason I have come. Chika's medical condition. He nods now and then, although I'm not sure he understands. "Whatever you think is best," he says, "you do."

I explain that her life could be in the balance.

"God will decide that," he says.

I say I have a hard question. I say if Chika should not survive this brain tumor, is it important to him that she be buried here in Haiti? I hate even saying the words, it makes me physically shiver, but it feels like something I must ask him. Perhaps he would want to visit her grave.

"It doesn't matter," he says. "Whatever you think."

I want to stoke a connection between father and daughter. It feels like I should try. Chika once said she had a memory of her father taking her for ice cream when she was very little. She said it made her happy.

Do you remember that? I ask Fedner.

"I never took her for ice cream."

Is there any place near here that sells ice cream?

"No."

I struggle to keep the conversation going. He is not mean. Just vacant. I keep thinking how sad it would make Chika if she heard there was no ice cream store.

Still, I invite him to the mission. I want him to see his daughter— and her to see him—perhaps because, deep down, I don't know if they will get another chance. We drive back together, and as we approach the gates, there is part of me that feels suddenly extrane-

ous, as if I've been nudged to the side of the picture. For all Janine and I have done with Chika, this man has a certain claim that we never will. It's different with her mother, who in dying, passed a torch that we eventually gripped. But Fedner Jeune is still here in Haiti. And while I force myself to ignore it, I feel strangely like a substitute.

When we arrive, Chika is playing in the gazebo. She is sweating heavily.

"Chika," I ask, "do you know who this is?"

She looks up.

"It's your daddy. Can you give him a hug?" (I say this in English so as not to embarrass him.)

She does as I ask. I leave them alone.

He sits on a bench, wearing a long-sleeved shirt, despite the heat, and she sits next to him. From time to time I look over, but I never see them speaking. Chika is playing with a doll and he is staring at the yard. The sun bakes down. One of our kids runs past with a "kite" made of sticks and a plastic bag, but with no wind, it doesn't take off.

After two hours, Fedner walks over, shakes my hand, and leaves.

Lesson Five

———

WHEN CHILDREN ARE YOURS AND NOT YOURS

We had a little boy in our orphanage for three years. He was sweet and well adjusted. One day, a man claiming to be his father came to our gate. He said he wanted the boy right now. We'd never seen this man before. The mother had told us during the intake interview that the child's father disappeared as soon as she'd gotten pregnant.

Now here he was, six years later, screaming threats at our director. When we contacted the mother, she begged us to ignore him. He was a violent person, she said, who just resurfaced and only wanted the child to prove dominance over her. She said her son would never go to school, or eat well, or be sheltered properly if we acquiesced. Please, she begged us, don't give him up.

A week or so later, she called and recanted. Crying and clearly distressed, she said the man was beating her, and if we didn't comply with his wishes, she was afraid for her life.

I told Alain we shouldn't do it. We couldn't do it. We'd be putting the boy—and his mother—in danger. I yelled and paced and yelled some more.

But in the end, we had no choice. There was no abuse hotline in Haiti. No court that would rule in our favor. The biological father had his rights. They trumped ours. It caused us great anguish, watching this boy play with the other kids, unaware of how his life was about to be uprooted. We pushed the deadline as long as possible, then reluctantly gathered his things. The nannies hugged him tightly. He started to cry. We drove him to an office, where, upon arrival, the angry father grabbed him without a word.

We never saw them again.

For three years our staff had fed, clothed, bathed, taught, and watched over that child. But the absent father's claim was greater, and we had to stand down. After that, we insisted on signed consents or death certificates for both parents in the intake process. But to this day, I agonize if that little boy is all right.

Yours, not yours. We wrestled with this question many times, Chika. Remember what you once asked? *How did you find me?* I promised myself you would never feel lost again. I hated the idea that you—or any of our kids—might ever feel unwanted.

But seeing your father that day touched a nerve. True, we

had to track him down. And he left the mission almost as quickly as he entered it. But what if he hadn't? What if he had said, "I'll take it from here"? Would I have been able, given your medical situation, to turn you over? To trust a man who had been so absent from your life to suddenly try and save it? Would I have been doing right by you? What about doing right by him?

Is it like Pope John XXIII once said, that it's easier for a father to have children than for children to have a real father? Who steps aside? It's a debate that foster parents deal with regularly and why adoption agencies have strict rules on parental rights. But we were neither of these. We were—we are—a place of love and shelter for Haitian children with few options. And when your health was threatened and we brought you to Michigan, and you were lying on that hospital gurney with tubes and monitors and a white bandage around your little head, who had claim to you was the furthest thing from our minds.

So this was another thing you taught me, Chika, what "yours" means with children and what it does not. It is an important lesson, and why I put it on this list.

Occasionally, by the way, even friends would use the "yours" word. *"It's great what you're doing for a child that's not yours."* It stung me to hear it, and puzzled me to think there would be a difference in our efforts if somehow you had our DNA. I remember once we stood by a mirror, studying our reflections, and you held your arm up next to mine. I thought you were comparing our skin color. Instead, you pointed to a mole near my wrist and said, "Mister Mitch, why do you have that bump?" That's all you were interested in.

Yours, not yours. The paperwork at the orphanage is signed by me. It obligates us to nurture, feed, educate, and protect the children—all things mothers and fathers are supposed to do. But in the end, it is a document of responsibility, not parenthood. I am, for all our kids, just Mr. Mitch, their "legal guardian," the words I used at the first hospital you and I went to, Chika. It feels sometimes like a diminished title. Still, when I look around, it is me, or Miss Janine, or our compassionate staff at the mission, kissing the children good night, waking them every morning, tying their shoes, cutting their sandwiches, reading them books, racing them to the doctor if something happens.

We did not bring any of these little souls into the world. That truth can never be overstated. But recently, one of our oldest kids, for whom we arranged a college scholarship in the U.S., honored a request to see his biological father in Haiti, who had never been a part of his life. The man quickly dragged him to his friends and bragged, "Look at my son! He's so smart he's in American college!" The young man said it made him resentful, as if this person, despite a lifelong absence, deserved credit for how he'd turned out.

I wonder, Chika, if anyone has blind claim over a child, save for God. I have witnessed the purest connection between an adoptive mother and her children, and I have witnessed helpless infants shunned by those who birthed them. The opposite also happens. After a while, you make peace with the truth: love determines our bonds. It always comes down to that.

The day your father returned home to Tabarre, you ran a high fever, and you vomited again. And that night, while he slept in his cinder block house, you cried yourself to sleep at the mission. The next day, you seemed so weak, that when the time came to leave, you didn't even say goodbye to the kids. You just took my hand and led me to the car.

At the Port-au-Prince airport, you complained about walking, so I carried you through the lines, one arm tucked beneath you, one arm wheeling my roller bag. When we boarded the plane, I put a pillow on the armrest.

"Go to sleep, sweetheart," I said, softly.

You lay your head down. After a few seconds you mumbled, "Mister Mitch?"

"Yes, Chika?"

"What will you do while I sleep?"

"I'll read," I said. "And think about how much I love you."

You nodded, your eyes glazed.

"That's what I'll do, too."

At that moment, I didn't care about who belonged to whom. I was yours, even if you were not mine. And as I stroked your forehead, which was hot to the touch, I knew I always would be.

Five

———

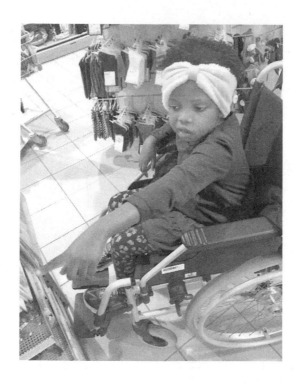

Us

———

The New Year passes with no visit from Chika. I go to Haiti for the holiday, as I always do, and we celebrate by lighting sparklers and singing "Auld Lang Syne" and the kids write resolutions on notebook paper that I slide into an envelope. (*"I will help clean the yard"* . . . *"I will not talk in class."*) We will open it twelve months later and see how they fared.

A special dish is served on New Year's Day, *soup joumou*, a pumpkin-tasting delicacy made from winter squash, potatoes, vegetables, onions, garlic, and pieces of beef. The soup was forbidden for slaves in the late-1700s, and is consumed on January 1 as commemoration of the Haitian revolution that established independence in 1804. Across the country, no matter how impoverished, families sip this soup as a proud tradition, a literal taste of freedom. Some of our kids are old enough to understand this. The younger ones are just happy with the soup.

Every night, when devotions end, we sing a song to remember Chika. It's the "L-O-V-E" song by Nat King Cole, which she used to belt out around the house. The kids sing it loudly, too, spelling along with the lyrics, clapping when the song says that V is very, very—*smack!*—extraordinary. At the end of the melody, they yell together, "One—two—three, good night, Chika!"

That night I go into the little girls' room. Chika's bed is still empty. The last time they saw her was that clipped visit when her fever and vomiting left her a shell of herself. She never returned. Maybe it was a blessing. Kids and farewells are a difficult mix.

When I get back to Michigan, it is snowing outside, and in the morning, I get a fire going in the fireplace. I turn to see Chika crawling out from under my desk, wearing blue shorts and a red-and-white-striped T-shirt.

"Arrrrrgggghh!" she yells, making tiger claws with her hands.

Good morning, beautiful girl, I say.

"I was trying to surprise you!"

You did.

"Then why you didn't scream?"

Sorry, I say. What were you doing under there, Chika?

"Oh." She studies her fingers. "You know. Looking."

Looking for what?

She exhales and lifts her eyebrows.

"Fairy doors! What else?"

———

Mott Hospital had fairy doors. We knew this from our many visits there, including the one we had to make the day after Chika and I got home from Haiti. She was hot, listless, short of breath, so we drove her to the emergency room of a hospital near us, but after checking her blood counts and several other tests, a doctor there confessed to not being familiar with the drugs Chika was taking, and suggested we go quickly to Mott's, where they knew her case.

"This could be something serious," the doctor said.

Janine cried in the ambulance as I followed in a car out to Ann Arbor; we spoke via cell phone the entire way. "They said it could be sepsis," Janine whispered.

"We don't know," I said, trying to stay calm.

As it turned out, the entire problem, and the reason Chika dragged through her final visit to Haiti, was a blood infection—caused by the port that the medical team had insisted upon. Somehow, bacteria had infected that port during Chika's one and only transfusion with it.

As a result, she spent nine straight days in a hospital bed, fighting a raging fever and tested for everything from meningitis to tuberculosis. A lung nodule had them concerned for a septic embolism. Her antibiotics were switched and switched again. Lab cultures were grown and studied. All because of bacteria that entered her bloodstream through what Janine would forever call "that stupid port"—which, of course, was taken out of Chika immediately.

"I never wanted that thing," Janine grumbled.

I felt as if she were blaming me.

"What were we supposed to do?" I said.

"Nine days she's been here, Mitch. Look how weak she's gotten."

"But they couldn't get a vein!"

She turned away.

"What were we supposed to *do*?" I yelled.

Janine and I argued more the worse Chika got. No surprise. It is hugely stressful, grappling with a child's illness, wondering if you are making the right moves. You feel lost. Uncertain. One of you can feel confident when the other doesn't, and you get angry at the difference. Half the time we were arguing to convince ourselves there was hope.

It found its way into little things with Chika. I would think some activity was safe; Janine would say it wasn't. I'd think a TV program was OK to watch; Janine would not. We bickered over antibiotics, nutrition. Janine would say, "I don't want her trying that" and I would say, again, "What are we supposed to do, nothing?" I think it all came down to the same thing: a fear of making the wrong move, or missing the right one. A fear of what was coming next.

It pained Chika to watch us disagree. She only wanted harmony. She would interrupt us by shouting, "OK-OK-OK-OK!" and waving her hands like a referee.

Then came a night when she was in the hospital, and

Janine and I were both upset over something. I was shaking my head, angrily repeating, "I can't *believe* this."

Chika called out from her bed, "What are you guys *talking* about?"

"Nothing, Chika," I said. "Don't worry."

"But it sounds *saaaad.*"

I walked over to her. "Yeah, sometimes things are sad in our lives, and sometimes things are happy. Like you. You're a happy thing. You make us happy."

She saw the frustration in my face, and began to tear up.

"Why are you crying, Chika?"

"Because," she whispered, "I don't know how."

"You don't know how to what?"

"To make you happy now."

That was the last time we spoke of such things in front of her. And the beginning of Janine and I realizing, in the end, we only had each other. We'd read where many couples eventually divorce after losing a child. We were determined to stay off that path. It's what ended disagreements before they got too wounding. One of us would mumble "I'm sorry, OK?" and the other would say "Yeah, I'm sorry, too" and we'd both exhale and steel ourselves for what came next.

By the time we took Chika home from Mott Hospital, her fight to stave off the infection had taken its toll. Her walking was worse. Her speech was slower. And she had a new partner, a PICC line catheter that came out of her right arm, through which her drugs and blood tests could now pass. We had to feed antibiotics, three times a day, through that line. It was covered with a little cloth sleeve and could not get wet, which meant showering was delicate, and swimming, which Chika loved to do, was off the table. It was summer, pool time, and that seemed so unfair.

Chika was just relieved to get home. She returned to her bed in front of ours. On her first morning back, Janine got up and lay beside her, and they started whispering, and pretty soon they were talking about Chika's favorite subject: weddings. Janine asked Chika where she thought she'd meet the boy she would marry.

"A restaurant," she answered.

I chuckled at her imagination. Then I realized Janine and I had met at a restaurant. We'd told her that once. Chika. Honestly. She remembered everything.

But all right. The fairy doors. They are little wooden portals, maybe six inches high, tucked into baseboards of various places in Mott Hospital. When you open them, there is a cartoon painted inside. Tinker Bell. A princess. People are encouraged to leave coins, so that a young patient might be surprised when he or she pulls open the tiny handle.

Chika was obsessed with finding these doors. She insisted on looking while still connected to an IV. Once I knew where a door was, I would sneak ahead—telling her I was looking for the fairies—and put a dollar bill behind each one.

"Look, a thousand dollars!" Chika would say, when she pulled the door open. (We never really taught her about money.) She'd put the bill in my hand, then start looking for another.

Watching her on that optimistic search, and passing rooms where I glimpsed parents with their heads in their hands, I realized something important: Hope is critical. It is almost mandatory to soldier through troubled times. Conversely, there is no affliction like hopelessness. I believe it is worse than anything that strikes the flesh.

We could not shield Chika from the tumor, or the pain, or even her own mortality. But we tried to project an aura of positivity, that we—the doctors and the nurses—all knew what we were doing, that life was still full of undiscovered treasures. Hopelessness can be contagious. But hope can be, too, and there is no medicine to match it. Chika's believing in us helped us believe in ourselves.

Surely there is a future, and hope will not be cut off. That's from Proverbs. We tried desperately to live that way, to believe in something good on the other side of all the little doors Chika opened.

———

"Mister Mitch."

Yes?

"Where are *your* fairy doors?"

We don't have them here. They're only at the hospital.

"Nuh-uhhh."

You saw them someplace else?

"Lots of places."

Like where?

She rests her elbows on my knees and taps her index finger against her cheek. She must have seen this in a movie, a sign that a person is thinking.

"Germany," she says.

"Children are not a distraction from more important work.
They are the most important work."

—DR. JOHN TRAINER

You

―――

Well. Since you brought that up.

There was much we didn't tell you about your medical journey, Chika. Research. Phone calls. Videoconferences. We were determined to shield you from the morass, but as anyone who cares for a sick child will attest, finding a cure consumes your every thought. You stay up nights wondering where else to look, and rack your brain in case you might be missing something.

To this end, the Internet is both the best and worst invention in the world. It has become, for people fighting serious illnesses, a seductive, confusing, often maddening place, a raucous bazaar of hope and horror. The wrong search word will pull up sites and stories you don't want to read, wild claims, heartbreak, accusations of fraudulent medicine, and countless entries beginning with the word *What*—"*What are the causes . . .*" "*What are the treatments . . .*" "*What are the signs . . .*" All you want to see is "*What is the cure?*" But it is never that simple.

I have read where years ago, Native American healers would rarely speak about their knowledge, or, in some cases, even identify themselves, so precious were their skills considered. The Internet is the opposite of that. You can find a thousand theories, contact a thousand practitioners, and never have the confidence you are not heading down a rabbit hole.

Early in your journey, Chika, I avoided the Internet for exactly these reasons. But after your blood infection, we needed to be more vigilant, to look beyond convention. You were already taking Panobinostat, the histone deacetylase inhibitor drug, because a Stanford doctor had seen some promise with it in mice. You'd endured a second round of radiation therapy, a risky, targeted approach, because that had been the only thing to deliver tangible results. We tightly controlled your diet. You drank your daily shake of supplements, even as you made a face while swallowing it.

But we were running out of vines to swing from. By this point we had come to know many DIPG cases. They often followed the same sad road map. Radiation. Chemo. A turn for the worse. A funeral.

Looking for an alternate story, we plunged, reluctantly, into the world of the Web. I read everything. Clinical trials. Facebook posts. I made calls overseas.

A program in London considered you, then said your progression and previous treatments "disqualified" you, a uniquely awful word, *disqualified*, as if you had broken some rule so you don't get to be cured.

They did, however, suggest a Belgian doctor working in Germany who was open to cases like yours. He specialized in immunology. And he was focused on DIPG.

His name was Stefaan Van Gool. I contacted him via email and he got right back, and Miss Janine and I had a long Skype conversation in which he answered many questions. He seemed a brilliant man, and was affable, kind, a father of four girls with whom he played violin in classical music concerts. Most importantly, he spoke about treatments we had not heard of in America—a vaccine made of the patient's own white blood cells and tumor antigens, to produce an immune system response that hopefully allowed it to attack the cancer. Our Michigan doctors didn't know of his practice.

"But if you think it will help, you should go," they said.

And so, as autumn began, and the kids at the Haiti mission went back to school, we booked airplane tickets and rented an apartment in Cologne, Germany, four thousand miles from our home. Sixteen months into your prognosis—and nearly a year longer than the doctors thought you would live—you were headed for yet another strange and new country, Miss Janine on one side, me on the other.

———

I want to speak about joy.

When I look back on our journey, there were times we didn't give enough weight to it. In the later stages, your daily needs were so great. Dressing you took longer. Bathing you was a meticulous process. Your PICC line needed to be flushed and kept sterile. Lifting and carrying you required me or someone else always to be present.

Because of this, we sometimes overlooked the fact that, despite the physical challenges, your mind kept growing. Your thoughts deepened. And we might have missed the joy of your blossoming into a fully formed young person—had you not made sure to reveal it in unique linguistic ways.

One time I was reading a long email, and I sighed and mumbled, "Oh, boy."

"Why do you say, 'Oh, boy'?" you asked. "There are no boys here."

"It's just an expression, Chika."

"Why don't you say, 'Oh, girl'?"

Another time, you asked for a glass of water. I warned you it was cold.

"Cold water, warm heart," you said.

(Where did *that* come from?)

You once asked Miss Janine, "Can I have two husbands?" And when she asked, "How many children do you want?" you shouted out, "One!"

"Why just one?"

"Because that's all I can CARRY!"

On a drive back from radiation, you asked, "Mister Mitch. Where are we going?"

I said, "Nowhere."

"Can we go nowhere together?" you replied.

And one morning, down in my office, my phone rang. It was you calling on the other line.

"Mister Mitch, do you want to come play fluffy, cozy bed camp?"

I entered the bedroom to find you and Miss Janine beneath the covers. When I crawled under, you said, "These are the rules of fluffy, cozy bed camp. I am the boss. Miss Janine is the second boss. You can be the third boss. Now. Let's play."

If I could change anything from those moments, Chika, it would be to stay in them a little longer. Immerse ourselves so we never forget. I rarely use the word *rejoice* in daily life, but it is the word I am looking for here. *Rejoice*. Revel in the funny business. It is quite something, when I look at photos of those days, to see your tireless crooked smile while miniature golfing, although you could barely swing the club, or on trips to the supermarket, although you had to sit in the basket, or a visit to the state fair, although I had to carry you from ride to ride.

No matter how engrossed we got in the medical struggle, you were indefatigable when it came to fun.

To paraphrase Emily Dickinson, because we could not stop for joy, you kindly stopped instead.

You awed us with your spirit.

She sits at the kitchen table, watching me.

"What are you doing?"

"I'm reading a book."

"What kind of book?"

"About Haiti."

"Why are you using that yellow thing?"

"I'm marking what's important."

"Mister Mitch?"

"Hmm?"

"Next time we go to Haiti, can I stay there?"

"You'll have to come back with me."

"Why?"

"We still have to see the doctors. You're still a little sick."

I say it quickly, without thinking. I don't realize this is the first time I have ever used the word sick with her.

"I'm not sick! I'm not sick!"

"OK."

"I'm just having trouble walking!"

You

———

When we landed in Germany, you met a new companion.

A wheelchair.

You gripped the handles. "This is for me?" you asked. I had to look away. Morrie, toward the end, was confined to a wheelchair. My mother, after her stroke, was, too. My father pushed her around for a year, until a stroke felled him as well, and he joined her in the seated world, the two of them draped by giant wheels, needing wide berths for passage.

For a stretch, we attempted to keep up their normal activities, going to movies, rolling them into restaurants, relying on home health care workers to lift them in and out of cars. But the world slowed down. Only certain places would accommodate us. I watched my parents sometimes, slumped back in resignation, tired shadows of their once energized selves. I could not put you in a wheelchair, Chika, without a choking in my chest.

But you, as usual, saw the world differently. You viewed that wheelchair as a faster way to get places, and for me to make it happen. We used that first one to maneuver through the Cologne airport, and out to a parking lot. With the cars zooming past us, you said, "Quick, Mister Mitch! Don't let them hit us!"

When we arrived at the flat we had rented, I carried you from the car, across the street, past a bus stop and through the front doors. When we got inside, we were greeted by two surprises:

An energetic Italian landlady named Antonietta.

And a long flight of steps.

"We have no lift here," Antonietta said, eyeing you in my arms. "I am sorry."

So, in addition to the wheelchair, our new routine included a series of up-and-down-the-staircase treks, with you clinging around my neck, piggyback style. There were nineteen steps. You weighed sixty pounds. So I was panting by the time we reached the top. You, of course, thought this was part of the fun, and crowed, "Mister Mitch, you need to sleep! You are tired!" I would get you inside the door, hurry you to the bedroom, and dump you on the bed, heaving air. By the time we'd get home, I'd be diagnosed with a hernia.

But you couldn't know that. Instead, you laughed, as if this whole trip was an adventure. It almost made us forget why we were there.

The clinic in Cologne was located on the fifth floor of a multipurpose office building, with a health club on the level below it and a supermarket next door. Unlike the hospitals in Michigan, there were no fancy lobbies, no high glass, no artwork or Superman statues. Just paneled hallways, narrow exam rooms, wooden desks, thin walls. We had to make K-turns with your wheelchair just to get around.

Still, the staff was kind, and Dr. Van Gool, wearing a white lab coat, was impressive in person. A highly respected Belgian immunology expert, he came to Germany, he said, because the doctor-patient laws there allowed him to more directly help needy children. He spoke many languages, and used English in academic ways that sometimes confused us. But there was a great warmth to him. He was short and chunky, with a sweep of straw-colored hair framing a high forehead and a jolly face, ruddy cheeks, and a long, horizontal smile. You liked him immediately.

"Zo," he began, as he began many sentences, "this is what we do. . . ."

What they did seemed brilliant in design. First they took a large sample of blood for the lab work. Then they infused you with something called Newcastle virus, a disease that is deadly to chickens but not dangerous to humans. The presence of the virus caused a response in the body's immune system, which they studied by removing cells after five days. The hope was that whatever defense your own body created, they could boost by loading the altered cells into the previously removed ones, then changing them in the lab, millions of them, then injecting them back into your body in a vaccine. The changed cells would, in theory, stimulate your immune cells to attack the DIPG tumor.

It was like training your own army to fight an enemy you created. Which is pretty much what cancer is.

Of course, to you, Chika, this was just something we did each day on the fifth floor. You took off your pink jacket and we lifted you onto the exam table. During the infusion, they stimulated the process with modulated electrohyperthermia, a round pad that pressed on your head and transmitted an electric field to your tumor area.

You never complained. Never asked why. You watched the movie *101 Dalmatians* on an iPad (you adored that film) until it was time to go.

Once, as we were leaving, you yelled "BYYYEEE!" to no one in particular from your wheelchair, and as we exited, I pressed the elevator button and you sang, "The SUN will come OUT, TOMORROW! . . ."

I could add more details about the immunology process, but what stays with me now, Chika, as I write these pages, is how happy you were in Germany. The flat was a far cry from our large house in Michigan. It was little more than functional: a small kitchen, a sitting room, a bedroom, and a bathroom in the middle. But you loved it. It was new, with blank white walls for your Magic Marker drawings. And it was yours. More importantly, we were yours. In Germany, the phone didn't ring. No one came to the door. I never went away to work. And all our little walking trips—to the clinic, to the market—we did together. Down the steps I would carry you, then position you in the wheelchair, lock the footrests, pull on the safety belt, and off we would go.

Cologne is quite beautiful, and in late September the sky was a brilliant blue. We rolled through the streets and the shopping plazas, and you sang so loudly, people turned as you passed. You sang anything that came to mind, "Blue Room" by Ella Fitzgerald, or "Santa Claus Is Coming to Town." We always told you to use your "inside voice" in the apartment, but here in the trafficked streets, you could belt to your heart's content.

We rolled down the pedestrian thoroughfare that led to the Kölner Dom, the famous, centuries-old Cologne Cathedral. The spires alone rise a tenth of a mile, pointing like arrows to the heavens.

"Oh, no!" you exclaimed when we came upon it.

"Oh, no, what?"

"Oh, no, I never see something like THAT before."

We both stared up, and you raised an arm against the sun. You were eating a piece of a Bavarian pretzel.

"Do you know what it is, Chika?"

"A princess castle?"

"No, it's a church. Where people pray."

"What do they pray for?"

"Well, I think they pray for everything. They pray for their family and they pray to get better if they're sick. They might be praying for you."

"They don't pray for *me*. I'm not their *child*."

"Well, you never know."

"But they don't even *know* me!"

"People don't have to know you to pray for you, honey.

They can just pray because you're a beautiful little girl and they want you to be healthy, right? And you can pray for them, too."

You nodded slowly, as if mulling it over, and you swallowed your pretzel and stared at the giant steeples.

"Wow," I mumbled.

"Wow," you repeated.

———

A word here about prayer.

The only photo we have from your infancy is of you being held up by a preacher at your baptism. You have the biggest smile, your eyes facing heaven. Perhaps that was a harbinger of your joyous faith.

Prayer was all over your young life. Your mother, I'm told, prayed along with the radio, and your godmother prayed constantly. At the mission, you and the kids prayed every morning and every night and every Sunday during church services. You would not eat before saying, *"God I thank you for this food I am about to receive . . ."* And before you fell asleep, you said the entire "Our Father."

So there was prayer wherever the day took you. But it was mostly ritual and gratitude.

The prayers of desperation were left to us.

One evening in Germany, to bless the food, you placed your hands together in front of you, and you closed your eyes, but your left eye couldn't shut at all. Eventually, at night, we had to put in drops, then tape that eye closed, so it wouldn't dry out.

You accepted this, because we said it was important. But such things, Chika, threw me to my knees. Watching you sleep with white tape over your eye? Your lying on a table as they drew more blood? My prayers were more like pleading. *Please, God, why does she have to go through this? Please, God, she's just a little girl.*

All during your time with us, I heard from people about "God's will" and "What God wants." I would like to tell you I accepted that without resistance, but if that were true, we might never have brought you to America for surgery, or fought against conventional treatment, or taken you to Germany. Was it God's will for you to be sick in Haiti, or God's will for you to be healed in a foreign country?

Miss Janine was better at this than me. So many times, I heard her in her room, or with friends or sisters, softly reciting, *"Heavenly father . . ."* She has always found comfort in prayer, and conversation with the Lord. For me, writing was more natural. When you write, you also feel like you are in conversation, and sometimes I wrote my thoughts down, as if God could read them, and I asked for strength.

But if prayer is supposed to bring peace, I could not always find it, Chika. I will admit that. I could not understand why a child had to suffer, why the Cologne clinic had so many kids needing help to walk or talk. This does not mean I lost my belief in God. But it was tested. C. S. Lewis, the man who wrote the Narnia books you so loved, once said it is easy to trust a rope as long as you're using it to wrap a box. But when you're clinging to it over a deadly precipice, it's something else entirely. As your condition worsened, my clinging became more desperate. I often got angry at the Lord.

The reason I didn't walk away altogether, I guess, harkens to something an old rabbi named Albert Lewis once told me. He had lost his four-year-old daughter to an asthma attack in the 1950s.

I asked if even he, a righteous clergyman, didn't get mad with God over that.

"Oh, I was furious," he said.

Then why didn't you stop believing?

"Because," he said, "as terrible as I felt, I took comfort in having something I could cry to, a power to whom I could shout, 'Why?' It is still better than having nothing to turn to at all."

That was the approach I took, Chika. At times I prayed, at times I howled and protested. Many times, I asked the Lord, "Why are You letting this happen?"

You never asked that. Your faith was pure. A child's often is. But that didn't keep you from occasional fear. One evening, you had trouble falling asleep. I sat by your bed and asked what was wrong. You said you were scared that the devil would come for you in the middle of the night.

"Don't be afraid," I said. "God is watching, so the devil can't get you."

You looked away.

"What if he comes when God's not looking?"

Six

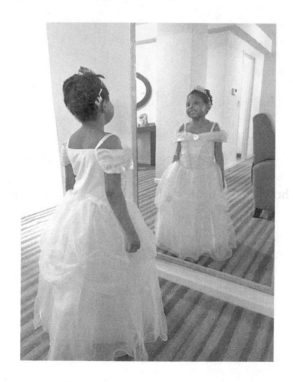

not sit so long

Me

———

As I write deeper into these pages, I find I am growing physically ill. My feet tingle. My hands get clammy. My head feels clogged and slightly dizzy. One morning, sitting at the keyboard, I begin to tremble, my pulse races, and I feel sweat beading on my forehead. My cheek goes numb. I wonder if I am going to pass out, or worse, suffer a stroke.

It happens several times. I visit doctors. Their tests come back clear. MRI. EKG. Blood work. I am told to hydrate more, drink less caffeine, get sleep. Perhaps not sit so long hunched over the screen, writing this story, as my spine and hips and neck are paying a price. But I continue to feel out of sorts, and sometimes my blood rushes and I feel as anxious as an accused man awaiting a jury.

Janine has her own diagnosis. "You're sitting there every day, revisiting a really hard time. It's emotional. You're grieving. You can't be surprised that your body is reacting to that."

"But why now?" I say, pushing back. "I made peace with all this already, didn't I?"

Janine looks at me as if I'm being naive.

"You loved her, Mitch."

That is all she says.

And that is what makes telling this last part so hard.

We had a routine about love, Chika and me. I'm not sure when it started. I would slide in front of her if she seemed sad, and I'd say, "Chika, have I told you today how much I love you?"

And, knowing what was coming, she would play coy.

"Nooo," she'd answer.

"This much!" I'd reply. And I'd stretch out my arms. With each passing week I'd stretch farther, because I knew she was measuring. In time, I advanced to hooking my arms behind my back, and spinning to show her my grip.

"Thissss muchhh," I'd warble, straining.

It brought a laugh, a satisfied laugh, because she knew I had gone the limit for her. She was always a little happier after that. A little calmer. And so was I.

I still remember the first time Chika said "I love you." It took a while. She would welcome the words from me or Janine, but she seemed in no rush to return them.

One night, when she had been with us maybe four months, I was in an airport and called home. Chika was energized. She enjoyed having Janine to herself. They were playing some sort of game.

"OK," I said at the end, "you be a good girl."

"I will," Chika said.

"I love you."

"I love you, too!"

I blinked and felt a rush of joy. I wanted to shout to Janine, Did you hear that? Did she really just say it?

But Chika hung up the phone, in a hurry to return to play-time, and I was left staring at the cell in my hands. It felt wonderful, just the same.

Us

———

"Mister Mitch?"

Hmm?

"We went to Germany three times."

That's right.

"I saw the zoo. And the bridge with all the locks."

She is talking about the *Hohenzollernbrücke* in Cologne, which straddles the Rhine river. Couples paint "love pad-locks" then snap them onto the bridge's gated wall to symbolize their commitment. There are more than forty thousand now. The weight is becoming problematic. Love, apparently, can at times be too heavy.

"Why didn't we go back again?"

To Germany?

"Uh-huh."

We couldn't.

"You mean *I* couldn't," she says.

I hesitate.

That's right, I say.

"Yeah." She makes a face. "I know."

She walks across the room, stopping at bookshelves to

examine their contents. It is cold and wintry outside, and this morning she appeared by running toward me from the office door, her feet making no sound on the carpet. I turned to see her last few steps before she rolled into a summersault, then landed on her bottom and yelled, "Yeeouch!"

I realize, watching her now, how much I studied Chika's walking during her time with us. Like her left eye and mouth, it was a barometer of her disease. I'd seen her stiff-legged when she first arrived, and unsteady after the surgery and steroids. I witnessed a return to almost normal after radiation, then a favoring of her left side as things declined.

Once, between trips to Germany, I saw her stomp away from us after growing angry over having to take some medicine. She yelled, "I DON'T WANT TO!" Then her legs gave way. She tumbled to the floor. I went to help her, but she pushed away and crawled to the bedroom steps. She pulled herself up one, slid down, then pulled herself up again. Chika surrendered many things during her battle with DIPG. Her will to fight was never one of them.

"Hey! Mister Mitch!" she says now.

I look up. She is holding the yellow pad. She points to the next-to-the-last item.

"Is this about Miss Janine?"

Lesson Six

———

WHEN A MARRIAGE BECOMES A FAMILY

Well, yes, Chika. I should have written about her sooner. But just as you were a revelation, so was what I learned about my wife.

Do you remember your first Thanksgiving morning with us? Miss Janine and I were in bed, talking. You pulled yourself up and crawled in closer.

"Are you going to work now, Mister Mitch?"

"Not today."

"Are you going to write a book?"

"Not today."

"Do you have to go somewhere?"

"Nope. I'm gonna stay here with you."

You looked away.

"Don't you *want* me to stay here with you?" I asked.

"Yeah . . ."

"But?"

"Um, don't you have to go to work or something?"

Miss Janine laughed. She knew you wanted to snuggle with her, and you needed me to clear out.

I was proud of how you tried not to hurt my feelings. But as I got up to make some coffee, I looked back and saw the two of you, already entangled, pulling up the covers, and I felt something else, something big and warm and satisfying. Your bond with Miss Janine had grown so naturally, it was hard to remember when it wasn't there. But it changed her.

And it changed the two of us as well.

Before you came to America, I kept updating Miss Janine. *Chika may need help. Chika may need surgery. Chika may need to stay with us.* I realize now I never asked if that was OK with her. And she never made me feel as if I had to.

That is no small thing. This is her home as much as it is mine. But she opened her arms the minute you arrived. And you found, in that embrace, something I could never give you.

It was Miss Janine who bathed you, and Miss Janine who dressed you. It was Miss Janine who picked out your Mary Jane shoes and helped you with the clasp. It was Miss Janine who put clips in your hair and whose hand you took when you marched toward the shower and yelled back at me, "Privacy, please!" When, out of the blue, you asked, "If I get married and I have to go potty, who is going to help me out of my wedding dress?" It was Miss Janine who said, "I will."

It was Miss Janine who sat and painted rainbows with you, and who made you blender drinks of supplements and got you to drink them. It was Miss Janine who soothed you if you wet the bed and were too embarrassed to tell me. It was Miss Janine who read you Bible verses and reviewed your schoolwork and who slept in the room your first night in a hospital. It was Miss Janine's long, dark locks that you liked to brush and pull over your head, as you leaned in and squealed, "Look, Mister Mitch! We have the same hair!"

When you did that, she would laugh and hug you close, and I'd be reminded again of how foolish I had been in the early years of our marriage, when I worried about having children. Men often fear that once they start a family, their wives will focus more on the kids, and their relationship will dwindle into car pools, chores, and laundry. This is based on something pretty childish in itself: an unwillingness to share attention.

But seeing you and Miss Janine together only left me more fulfilled. You think you know your spouse after so many years together, and I thought I knew Miss Janine completely. I knew her moods and what moved her, I knew her sounds and her looks. I knew that she was warm to strangers and loved her family fiercely, and had a razor wit and was an amazing singer who often felt too shy to demonstrate how good she was. I knew she loved fresh bread, calamari, the Beatles, gospel singing, and having everyone over the house, crashing on couches. I knew she often had joint pain, which she endured quietly, that she couldn't hang up on telemarketers, that the death of her older sister Debbie was a mountainous tragedy in her life. I knew she gave everyone in her world, no matter what harm they'd done, a second and a third chance.

And I knew she loved me more than I deserved, took my side in any conflict, and would still, after twenty-seven years together, sound excited when I called her on the phone.

But your arrival, Chika, triggered something new, a sense of discovery that happens for most couples, I guess, much earlier than it did for us. It was a splash of new color on an otherwise familiar canvas. Watching her dress you, bathe you, nurture you, sing to you, gave me a deeper appreciation for this woman whom I married, and her instincts that were coming now so easily to the fore, like a bud that had been waiting decades for sunshine.

That first Thanksgiving, you wanted to dress up, so she outfitted you in a sparkly blue tutu and a little black sweater, with a headband that featured a large pink flower. You asked to wear a necklace and she gave you two, and you looked in the mirror, so proud of yourself. I don't know where your penchant for fashion came from, Chika, but I suspect you'd often watched Miss Janine get dressed, and in some way, you wanted to be like her.

That night we made a toast to the new faces at the table. Miss Janine said how grateful we were to have you with us. For the first time in countless Thanksgivings, we felt less like a couple and more like a family. I know how much that meant to her.

By your second Thanksgiving, after two trips to Germany, things had changed so much. Your speech was slowed. Your eye drooped severely. You weren't able to run or play with the other kids. Eating was a laborious process. You drooled food sometimes. Worst of all, for you, Aidan seemed more interested in the other cousins, who were racing around the house. When we sat you two together to eat, you didn't have much to say. Maybe you felt self-conscious. When the meal was over, he ran off to play.

Miss Janine and I saw the hurt in your eyes. Sitting on the couch, you asked us, "Why doesn't Aidan love me?" I wanted to grab the boy and make him stay next to you all night. But Miss Janine was more tender in her answer. She told you not to worry, that all things come in time, and that you were beautiful and she was so proud of you. And I was never prouder to be her husband.

There were moments when you wanted to call Miss Janine "Mommy." It touched her heart, more than you know. But as much as she might have privately desired that, she always reminded you of who your mother was, and was always seeking out information to share with you.

One night you were watching the movie *Pan*, a scene where Peter Pan sees a vision of his departed mom. When it ended, you asked if you would ever see your mommy again.

"Yes, sweetheart," Miss Janine answered. "You'll see her in heaven."

"But how will she *know* me?"

"Mommies never forget their babies."

You dropped your head. "But how will I know *her*?"

We realized your memories did not go back that far. In truth, you had been with us—at the orphanage and then in America—longer than you'd been with your mother or your godmother. Some might take that as a claim to the *Mommy* word. But Miss Janine was not concerned with titles, only with loving you, protecting you, and making you aware of all the wonders of this life, including who you were before you graced our little universe.

Remember how you fantasized about getting married, Chika? Well, when people get married, they share the love of a couple. But when children arrive, they create another love, not just for the new additions, but for the new entity they have created. The family. It is not better than a couple's love, it's complementary, forged with a new appreciation, and a wider, expansive heart.

I think back now on the three times a day, every day, Miss Janine cleaned your PICC line, slowly, studiously, rubbing the alcohol pads to insure no infections. I think about all the baths and toilet duties and dressing and undressing of you that she did. I think back on all the mornings the two of you played under the covers, all the movies where you sat in her lap, all the times she let you brush her hair, or try on her earrings, or lead her by the hand to whatever new discovery you just *had* to show her, saying "Miss Janine! Look!" I think about her sitting beside you, long after you'd fallen asleep, praying for a miracle, then looking at me with tears in her eyes and whispering, "We can't lose her, Mitch. We can't."

There may be other words for that besides *Mother*, but it's as motherly a role as I know. And getting to see Miss Janine that way was a rare and precious gift. You showed it to me, Chika. That is why it's on the list.

One afternoon, we hear her singing from the bedroom. Janine gets a camera. It's a gospel song called "No Longer a Slave" that the kids in Haiti do in devotions. Chika is singing it verse after verse, sitting up in bed, wearing a yellow T-shirt and pajama pants.

Normally, when an adult enters a room, children will stop singing, especially if that adult is trying to film them. But when Janine enters, Chika doesn't stop. Her eyes are almost glazed, and she seems in communion with something invisible.

"I'm no longer a slave to fear
I am a child of God."

She sings it for eight minutes. Nonstop. Even with the camera inches away from her face. When she finishes, she lies down and closes her eyes.

Janine emerges from the room, stunned.

"She sang to herself all that time?" I ask.

"Not to herself," Janine answers. "She was talking to God."

You

———

Our final trip to Germany, in early December, felt a bit like coming home. Same apartment in Cologne. Same funny Italian landlady. Same nineteen steps. Same wheelchair rides to the markets, plazas, and clinic. And you, Chika, were happy to be away from the Thanksgiving crowd and back in the center of attention.

But it was colder, and we had to bundle you up tightly with blankets. Your speech was noticeably slower and your torso wobbled back and forth, which made it look like you were keeping a dance beat, but in truth was a slow loss of your motor control. When we ate, you had trouble pressing the knife down and you drank things through a straw so as not to drop the cup. At a Christmas market, I saw you studying your fingers, struggling to wiggle them one at a time.

There were other ominous signs. A young girl you had befriended at the clinic was not coming back, because her tumor had advanced and a second one had formed. One visit, while you watched a movie on an iPad, Dr. Van Gool showed Miss Janine and me statistics of his studies to date, graphs with black and green lines, green representing the newest patients. The goal, he said, was to get the green line to curve and flatten above the black, suggesting a truce between the immunology treatment and the DIPG progression.

Near the end of the black, I saw a string of red markings.

"What are those Xs?" I asked.

Miss Janine touched my arm.

"Those are crosses," she whispered. "It means they died."

That night, in the cramped kitchen of the flat, we played children's songs as you tried to color. You sang along as well as you could. You seemed to be rekindling a love of nursery rhymes, maybe because they were simpler to remember. You loved "Twinkle, Twinkle, Little Star."

I remember us in the backseat of a car once, singing that song, and you putting your hand over my mouth so you could finish solo. Afterward I asked, "Did you know you can wish upon a star?"

"Huh?"

"You can say 'I want to put a wish on that star and it will help my wish come true.'"

"Or," you suggested, softly, "we could make a star come to us."

"To us?" I said.

"Like a gift."

"You mean pull it out of the sky?"

"Yeah."

"And let it knock on the door and say 'Hello'?"

"Noooo . . . Stars can't talk."

I should have said, yes, Chika, they can, because I was listening to one. Instead I mumbled, "That sounds like a good idea," and you leaned your head into my chest and I kissed your hair. I could have stayed in that moment a long time, looking down at your cheeks and nose and eyes. We adults can be a wretched lot, Chika. Yet in every child's face we see the Lord has not given up on us. Yours was proof of that.

———

When we came home from Germany, something must have happened. You were sluggish. You threw up in the car. Your eyes lost focus. Your sentences started strong but trailed to a whisper.

We took you to Mott Hospital, where they did an MRI. The worst was confirmed. There was "significant progression" of the disease. I thought about how much that word had changed for us, *progression*, which used to mean something positive and now was anything but. Christmas hung on the calendar, a week away, Miss Janine had the tree up, and people were already dropping off your presents. Sometimes I caught you sitting on the floor, gazing at the ornaments, but you didn't say anything, and when I asked, "Whatcha looking at, Chika?" you stared at me before you answered, blinking, as if trying to find me in a snowstorm.

Us

"OK, I'm gonna go now."

Why, Chika?

"Because you're gonna get sad."

Is that bad?

"It's not bad. It's just . . ."

She taps her cheek with her finger again.

". . . not fun."

Do you only want to have fun?

She throws out her hands. "Ummm, yeah! I'm a *child*!"

She says *child* in two syllables, "chi" and "uld." I don't know how to respond.

"I'll come back when you are done," she says.

Wait! I shout.

She looks at me curiously.

Where do you go? When you're not here. Where do you go? Can you tell me? Can you tell me what it's like?

She looks down.

"Can *you* tell *me* what it's like?" she says.

This was something she often did when she wasn't sure of an answer. Affect a false confidence. Like the time she was

204

singing a show tune and stopped in the middle. Janine asked her, "Don't you know the rest of the words, Chika?"

"*I* know," she cooed. "But *you* don't."

No, I answer her now, I can't tell you what it's like. I want to believe that you are happy and at peace and with God and forever young. That you get to play and laugh and use every part of your body. Is that it? Is that what it's like where you go when you're not here?

She lifts on her toes.

"How come you don't feel good, Mister Mitch?"

What do you mean?

"You have lots of hurts."

I don't know, I say. The doctors can't find anything.

"Not those hurts."

She puts her hand on top of mine. Her T-shirt has drawings of ice-cream cones.

Please stay, I whisper.

"It's a hard-knock life!" she sings.

And she is gone.

Seven

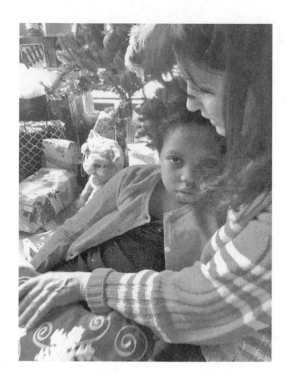

You

———

Do you remember a night in Germany, when we were all in the same bed, and you said to Miss Janine, "I have a secret to tell you"? And Miss Janine said, "What?" And you whispered, "Kiss Mister Mitch." So with you lying between us, we kissed over your head, and you said, "Now you can live happily ever after."

If only.

I didn't want to reach a seventh chapter in this book, Chika. I wanted to stop at six, like the A. A. Milne poem, be clever as clever, stay six forever. You were good at six. You had your funniest moments. Your biggest adventures. You were still six on our last trip to Cologne. I remember pushing your wheelchair past an elderly homeless woman sitting on the pavement. You asked what she was doing. I said she needs help and we should give her money. So you took the bills I handed you in an unsteady grip and you swayed as you leaned toward her. "Hi," you mumbled, and she smiled, the way you made everybody smile. And I thought, OK, Lord, we can stop here, we'll take this, even if she's in a wheelchair for the rest of her days, even if she sways, and mumbles. Please, just stop here and we'll be grateful.

But we don't get to set our stops.

For the record, the treatments we tried toward the end of your battle were vast and varied. We left nothing unexplored. We resumed the Avastin infusions at Mott Hospital. Meanwhile, at the suggestions of various doctors around the world (thank the Internet) we pursued something called peryllil alcohol, which you inhaled through a nebulizer, and later something called valproic acid, which was injected through your PICC line. We chased after a PMK inhibitor from a major drug company that matched a mutation in your tumor and, in theory, might have some effect, even though it wasn't designed for such use.

I doubt any of this means much to you, Chika, nor do the hours of debate, research, phone calls, hand-wringing, or flat-out begging to get our hands on some of these things, which was often difficult and contrary to conventional medicine. We kept this all away from you, and I believe that was the right choice. Still, I want you to know that we tried.

In writing these pages, I read your medical file provided by the hospital. I saw an entry in December of 2016:

Her neurological status has deteriorated acutely, with marked weakness/decreased tone (and) near absent/dysarthric speech. Her MRI corroborated further radiographic deterioration.

Nevertheless, her guardians continue to want to pursue active treatment. . . .

Nevertheless. That word stood out. You were now nineteen months into surviving something they thought would take you in four, and the word being used was *nevertheless*. It summed up the battle Miss Janine and I often felt we were fighting with the medical world. Because to doctors, no matter how empathetic, you were one of many, and to us you were one of one.

On another level, *nevertheless* was a perfect word. It means "despite anything to the contrary." And there was so much in our journey that was to the contrary, Chika, right from the start. We were unlikely to have encountered you in Haiti. You were unlikely to be in our care. We were too old. You were too young. The tumor was supposed to take you fast. We were supposed to accept that.

Nevertheless, here you were.

Nevertheless, here we were, too.

Me

———

I wonder if you know what's happening now at the mission, Chika. Are you able to see? Do you drop in there as you drop in with me?

Are you aware of the four new children who are sleeping in the little girls' room that you once called home? Or that Miss Anachemy, your wonderful former teacher, had a baby boy? Or that our older kids go with Miss Gina on Saturday mornings to hold infants at a clinic for premature babies?

Can you see the planting garden we began, right next to the school building, with kale and beans and spinach, that was protected by wire until one of the kids accidentally ran into it and knocked it down? Or the small music room we have now with a drum set and a couple of guitars and a little keyboard?

Do you hear Mr. Yonel, our second Haitian director, when he prays for you in the chapel on Sundays? Do you know that your two oldest mission brothers, Siem and Emmanuel, are now in America, on college scholarships? Did you see that when they moved into their dorm room and unpacked their simple belongings, they took out a picture of you and put it on the desk?

Are you aware that Emmanuel is studying to be a doctor, because he wants to help children after what happened to you? Can you see the influence you still have, even being gone? Is that a blessing bestowed on us when this life is over?

Or is it just a fierce and desperate hope we have on Earth, like the one we had about finding you a cure, something that remained forever beyond our control?

You

Your final Christmas was a muted one. We took you to the annual family gathering the night before, but you mostly watched as the other kids ate and opened presents. We were hand-feeding you by this time, spooning you soft foods, because your ability to hold utensils was shaky, and swallowing had become an issue.

The next morning, we had our own little holiday at the house, just the three of us. Miss Janine dressed you in a red sweater for the occasion, and we cradled you in our laps as you opened gifts. You swiped at the wrapping paper, determined to get through all of them, even as your arms swung out of control. You mumbled, "Wha' issit?" when the wrapping fell away, and I held up each new toy and explained it, waiting until you nodded.

It took most of the morning. There was no squealing or cheering, no racing to set up toys, no pancakes or eggs or toast with almond butter, because you could no longer eat such things.

But remember what I said about Christmas mornings

with no children? For the first time in our lives, that wasn't true for us, Chika. And for the first time in your life, you had a mother and father figure all to yourself on the holiday. That afternoon, sitting with you at the table, Miss Janine began to cry. With your hand wobbling, you reached for a tissue and gently patted her tears. Then you pushed our two faces together so we would kiss.

There were moments at this stage, Chika, when I wondered if we were pushing you too hard. If the treatments weren't wearing out your precious little body. The things you endured. The side effects. You often looked so weary.

But having you there that Christmas, in our arms, watching you unpack a red stocking, just knowing you'd made it to another day—and to this day in particular—felt full and lovely and very much like a family trying to cherish every moment, which is sometimes all a family can do.

Two weeks later, we celebrated your seventh birthday. For this event, everybody came. I mean everybody. Our sisters and brothers, our cousins, their kids, all your "friends" in their forties, fifties, and sixties, and the pied piper line of contacts you had made, from nurses to musicians. What a crowd you drew! We had it at our house, and we dressed you in your favorite yellow Belle dress, and when Miss Janine and several friends wheeled you into the room, I played "Happy Birthday to You" on the piano as the crowd sang along.

We'd arranged for two "princesses" to attend, dressed

as Cinderella and Sleeping Beauty, and when they came through the door, despite whatever heaviness your brain was feeling, you lit up. The princesses played games and gave out gifts and sang songs accompanied by a boom box, including "A Dream Is a Wish Your Heart Makes," which ends with the lines about grieving but believing, and your wish will come true. You couldn't really say much; you sat between Miss Janine and me most of the time, holding our hands. But your eyes followed everything.

I couldn't stop hugging you that afternoon, Chika, I'm not sure why. I'd walk away for a minute, then come back and lift you up, gathering the billowing yellow skirts under my forearms. Sometimes, I felt you burrow into my shoulder, and I tried to get you to look at your cake, but you couldn't lift your head. It was the happiest and most heartbreaking birthday I have ever experienced.

On my next trip to Haiti, I ask Alain to take me to a cemetery. He nods but says nothing. Nothing needs to be said.

We go to a place called Parc du Souvenir, with an entrance driveway that slopes up through big gates. It is quiet and hot when we get out of the car, and I see uneven rows of headstones in patchy grass, some of it green, some of it dried to the color of sand. The markers are so close together. I cannot imagine this for Chika. My breath accelerates. I am sweating.

A worker approaches and I ask him to show us a more secluded area. He says there is no such thing. We keep walking. The headstones are shaped like large white padlocks. Many of them have two, three, even four names.

"They bury people on top of each other," Alain says.

He sees my reaction.

"This isn't how you do it?"

The sun is brutal. I hear a truck go by. Several workers have now attached to us, one wearing garden gloves. They seem curious about an American doing the searching. We finally find a small corner, under some trees, where there are two unused plots together. I see a butterfly flitting between the tree leaves. I watch it fly away.

"*Can we get both of these?*" I ask Alain. "*So there can be more space?*"

"*We can ask,*" he says.

In the office, a middle-aged woman with glasses and crimson lipstick takes my information. When I tell her I want to buy the two plots, she says, "For how many people?"

"*One person. A child.*"

Her eyes bulge.

"*That does not make sense. You can bury ten people.*"

"*I understand,*" I say. "*But this is what I would like.*"

She shakes her head.

"*Maybe you will have other children who will need it?*"

I just look at her. What do you say to that?

She finishes the paperwork. I make the payment. We get back in the truck, and the man with the garden gloves waves as we exit.

It's a quiet ride back to the mission. Upon arrival, I see some of our kids playing soccer, and a few jumping rope. Two of our girls, about Chika's age, are leaning against a picnic table, looking at the sky, as if the hours will never run out. How can certain children have so much time, and Chika have so little?

I feel suddenly ashamed, like I just did something terrible. I want to race back to that cemetery and yell, "Cancel everything! A mistake has been made! She's just a kid!" But Alain has taken the truck to buy diesel fuel for the generator, and I am left there alone, standing in the sun.

Lesson Seven

———

WHAT WE CARRY

One afternoon, when you could no longer walk on your own, we were coloring at the kitchen table. I glanced at my watch and realized I was late. I stood up.

"Sorry, Chika, I have to go."

"No, no," you protested. "Stay and color."

"Chika, I have to work."

"Mister Mitch, I have to *play*."

"But this is my job."

"No, it's not!" You crossed your arms. "Your job is carrying *me*."

I have thought about that sentence more than you could imagine. At the time, I laughed it off as you being your lovable, bossy self. But the more you weakened, the more you needed me to transport you even across the room, the more I realized the wisdom of your words. *Your job is carrying me.*

That line became the underpinning of the final item on my list, maybe the biggest lesson you taught me.

What we carry defines who we are.

And the effort we make is our legacy.

The first week of February is traditionally Super Bowl week. For sportswriters, this is a big event. I had covered every Super Bowl since 1985. Thirty-two years straight. It was something my newspaper expected me to do, and I'd actually grown a bit proud of my little attendance streak, figuring I'd keep it up until I retired.

But I didn't go in 2017. All the things I had carried before, all the work that had once seemed so critical, had come to a halt, dumped out like a flatbed emptying its contents. When that week arrived, signaling your twenty-first month of battle—which put you on the furthest reaches of DIPG survival—you were in a different place than at your birthday party a month earlier. The tumor, as Dr. Van Gool put it, "had grown quite scandalous." You could no longer eat on your own, so a feeding tube had become necessary. At first, they tried one that went through your nose and down your throat. You yanked it out when no one was looking. (Honestly, part of me wanted to cheer you. Who would want such a thing?)

But that only led to a more stable version, a G-tube that was surgically placed inside your abdomen. Every day and every night we would load new bags of liquid food and run them through the stand-up pump, down the tube, and into your belly. We also infused medications through your PICC line multiple times a day, sterilized it, flushed it with heparin, tucked it under the small white sleeve on your arm. We nebulized the peryllil alcohol through a plastic tube in your nose.

I don't know how you handled it, Chika, all the apparatus. But even with all that, even with your precious voice reduced to a few grunted sounds, you were still you. You would dip your head ever so slightly to show me which doll you wanted to sleep with at night. You would wave a wobbly hello when we FaceTimed with the kids in Haiti. One time I was coughing badly, and your eyes turned to me, and Miss Janine said, "He needs someone to smack his back. Chika, do you want to hit Mister Mitch?" I leaned down, and you tapped me three times.

The day of the Super Bowl, I was sitting on your bed, flipping through movies for you to watch. I read the titles out loud and you didn't react until I came to *Mr. Peabody & Sherman*. You raised a thumb. So I watched it with you.

At one point in that movie, Mr. Peabody, a dog, goes before a judge to adopt his protégé, Sherman, a boy.

The judge asks, "Are you sure you're capable of meeting *all* the challenges of raising a human?"

And the dog says, "With all due respect, how hard can it be?"

———

I've decided, sitting here, that I will not explain in any great detail the final eight weeks we had with you, Chika. They were difficult and trying, with last-ditch medical attempts, and an oxygen machine, and rubber thumpers that we used on your back to get you to cough, and a suction tube that went in your nose and throat to pull up the stuff that was blocking your breathing. You wore a small monitor on your finger to measure your pulse and oxygen levels, and it flashed red numbers all through the night, waking Miss Janine and me with beeps if a level moved too high or low. It got to be that I knew the right numbers—and the wrong ones—within a second of my eyes opening. I don't hate many things, Chika, but I hated that monitor. It was like a glowing red countdown on your existence.

Still, there were positives. You continued to effuse a life force that melted the most experienced workers. A team of physical therapists from a place called Walk The Line started making house calls when you could no longer travel there, because, they said, "We miss Chika." A chief nurse named Donna from a company called Health Partners would drop by unscheduled, just to see how you were doing. There were times when I would walk in the room and you had two of our friends, three of our family members, a couple of health care workers, and someone playing the ukulele. You drew the biggest crowds.

One night we told a nurse named Shawn, who was tall like your mother, how much you liked church music. Out of the blue, she asked if she could sing for you.

And with all of us gathered around, and you lying in your

little medical bed, Shawn launched into the most beautiful rendition of "His Eye Is on the Sparrow."

"I sing because I'm happy
I sing because I'm free
His eye is on the sparrow
And I know He watches me."

Your eyes watched in wonder. And there was wonder in that moment. Miss Janine wept.

Your final days took us into April, when the clocks had been pushed forward and the weather had warmed. You had now made it to a twenty-third month. That is exceptionally long for someone with DIPG. Miss Janine had said you were a miracle, and in so many ways you were.

I studied you each evening before turning out the lights, so still, so innocent, your lineless face without expression. It's hard for me to explain how helpless I was feeling, Chika, unable to fight beside you in whatever battle was raging in your head. How were you so strong? I thought about the tale of Jacob and the angel, wrestling by a riverbank all through the night. I've often wondered why that fight took so long, since the angel only had to touch Jacob's hip to cripple him.

But I suppose it was Jacob's fierce determination that brought him to the morning light. And it was your fierce determination, Chika, that brought you to this point, still here, after nearly two years of wrestling.

Yes, the price was dear. We lost your lovely voice along the way, and had only your half-open eyes, into which I would look each day and say, "Good morning, beautiful girl." Your body, through so many weights and changes, had returned to the thin, long-legged form of your arrival in America. You were taller by a few inches, but in certain ways, you had come full circle.

In the predawn hours of April 6, your numbers dropped precipitously. Your heartbeat was way down, and your breaths came sporadically. I was sleeping on the floor by the closet, because the beeping monitor had kept me awake, when I heard a hospice nurse call my name. I sprung up in the darkness, shouting, "What? What?" and the nurse said, "It might be time."

Miss Janine and I leaned into you, rubbing your soft cheeks. We tried to steel ourselves. But as the morning broke in a gray fog, it did not feel right. It did not, to us, feel like "time." I pushed my ear against your chest and I heard a sound, almost a groaning.

"She's struggling," I said.

"Those are just the sounds children make," one of the hospice workers said, "at the end."

I looked at Janine. She shook her head. I felt the way I did in that conference room with Dr. Garton two years earlier.

"No," I said. "She's fighting. And if she's fighting, we're fighting."

I leaned you forward, and, forgive me, Chika, if I did the wrong thing, but I began pounding on your back with the small rubber thumpers, as I had been taught, and running the suction tube through your nostrils and down your throat, as I had been taught, and pounding again, saying, come on, baby, come on, baby, if you want to fight, then fight. And with the hospice workers watching in utter astonishment, your heartbeat lifted and your respiration increased and within five minutes you were back to a safe zone. Miss Janine stared at me, both of us heaving breath, and one of the hospice workers whispered, "I've never seen that before."

And through our tears, Miss Janine and I thought of the same word:

Nevertheless.

What you carry is what defines you. It can be the burden of feeding your family, the responsibility of caring for patients, the good that you feel you must do for others, or the sins that you will not release. Whatever it is, we all carry something, every day. And for all your time with us—as you so defiantly stated, Chika—my job was carrying you.

My job was—and is—carrying your brothers and sisters in the orphanage.

My job, it turns out, after so many years without them, is carrying children.

It is the most wonderful weight to bear.

One night, while she can still speak, Chika takes a small stuffed bear to bed. A gift from the hospital. A Care Bear, they call it.

The bedroom is dark. I kneel down next to her.

"Well, hello," I whisper to the bear. "Do you belong to Chika?"

Chika puts the bear in front of her face.

"Yes," she murmurs.

"You're a lucky bear. I think Chika is a really special girl."

"Uh-huh."

"But don't tell her. That's between you and me."

"I am Chika's bear," she says, "so I have to tell her everything."

"Well, don't tell her how much I love her. It's a secret."

"Chika already knows how much you love her."

"She does?" I say, skeptically. "How much?"

Chika takes the arms of the bear and does what I always do, pulling them around until they touch behind its back.

"Thiiisss much."

My eyes tear up.

"That's right," I whisper. "That much."

You

And so.

After you rallied so brilliantly on that foggy April morning, we called everyone who loved you, and everyone you had touched, and we told them if they wanted to see you, they should come see you now. And they did. Oh, my, they did. You loved a parade? Well, you had one of your own, Chika, a day-long procession of family, friends, and your small army of touched souls. They came and sat by you, holding your hands, and we shared the details of that morning's return from the brink. And if that was the final story in the million or so we have told of you, it was a good story, a brave and defiant one, which is what you were.

That night, all the kids from Haiti were gathered after devotion, and we held an iPad up to your ears as each of them said, "Good night, Chika" or "Good night, precious."

The next day, April 7, was a fine spring morning. And just after lunchtime, with the sun up high like an island sky, you began to say goodbye.

This time there was no horror, no bolting up in the darkness, no groaning sounds. You were lying on your back, your head tilted down. There was soft Haitian music playing. Miss Janine got in one side of your bed, I got in the other, and we held you, the way you liked, the way we did in Germany when you told us to kiss and live happily ever after. Someone had figured out how to put photos on the bedroom TV, and they flashed silently, happy photos of your time here, wearing your swimming goggles, playing with me in a sandbox, slurping ice cream. There you were, a few feet away, untouchable, yet so full of life. And here you were, just inches away, so touchable, yet slipping from this world.

"We love you, Chika," I repeated, softly. "We love you so much . . ."

We rubbed your fingers. Your shoulders. Your cheeks, which, to the end, had a softness we have never found anywhere else on Earth. We kissed you many times. We counted your breaths. They came so slowly. Only five in a minute.

Then four.

Then three.

It got very quiet. Family and friends waited outside. It was just the three of us entangled together, like the fluffy, cozy bed camp you created and loved.

Finally Miss Janine, tears dripping down her cheeks, took a deep breath and whispered, "It's all right now, Chika. . . . You can go be with your mommy in heaven."

Finding Chika

She broke down, sobbing, and my heart snapped in two, because I knew how hard that was to say.

And I knew that you would listen to her.

Two breaths.

One.

Finding Chika

She broke down, sobbing, and my heart snapped in two, because I knew how hard that was to say.

And I knew that you would listen to her.

Two breaths.

One.

Us

———

My head is in my hands. My eyes are bleary. I feel like I am going to pass out.

"It's finished?" Chika says.

I barely look up.

It's finished, I say.

"See? I said I would come back."

I rub my cheeks with my palms.

Come here, sweetheart, I say.

She steps in front of me. She has the My Little Pony pajamas on again, her hair is tightly braided, and she looks like the first morning she woke up in our house, and we made scrambled eggs together.

Listen, I say, choking up. I know this is all in my head. I know you can't really be here in front of me. But I want to tell you something while you are.

"Ooookay . . . ," Chika drones, placing her elbows on my knees and resting her face in her palms. "What do you want to say?"

Just this. You weren't my child. But you were my child to me. I could not have loved you more, and Miss Janine could not have loved you more. And wherever you went after you left this earth, you went as part of a family, actually, a lot of families. You made us a family, Chika. Miss Janine and me and you. I wish more than anything that we could have saved you, even if the Lord had different plans. But we miss you every minute. And you never have to worry about us forgetting you, because we could never forget you, we'd lose every memory we ever had before we would let go of yours. You took a huge part of us with you, Chika, the best part, but it was yours to take, and I hope it will always be close to you. I just wanted to say that, in case, for even a fleeting second, you thought you left this world alone.

She scrunches her lips, as if thinking. Then she grins and throws open her arms.

I reach out—and for the first and only time, I can initiate contact, I can touch her again. I pull her in, I feel her forearms around my neck, her soft cheeks and braided hair against my temples. I snuggle her into a familiar embrace, and she fits as if she never left.

She leans back, smiles, and pulls her pajama top over her head.

"Where is Chika?" she asks.

She puts her hand against my heart.

"There she is!"

And she is gone.

Epilogue

———

Medjerda "Chika" Jeune was buried in Haiti on the fifteenth of April 2017. Many of the Americans she touched flew down for the ceremony, which was also attended by her god-mother, her father, the entire staff of our orphanage, and, to our surprise, her younger brother and two older sisters. A small group went to the grave site afterward, where butter-flies flitted around the trees that shaded her corner.

On her grave marker were the words from the song she sang by herself that night:

MWEN SE PITIT BONDYE
"I am a child of God."

Later, back at the orphanage, our kids gathered in their best clothes for their own little church ceremony. Many of them stood and declared their favorite thing about Chika, including "she really liked to eat." After that, we released three dozen pink balloons in her honor, and they lifted into the air and flew over the streets of Port-au-Prince.

As I moved around the grounds, I spotted her baby

brother, Moïse, and I almost lost my breath. He looked so much like her. He was three years old, the same age as Chika when she came to us. I offered him a hug and he jumped into my arms and squeezed me with a grip that was new and old at the same time.

Later that afternoon, his guardian, Chika's uncle, asked to speak to me. He said he had taken Moïse after Chika's mother died because the child had no place else to go. But he and his wife had children of their own, and money was hard to come by. He saw the mission facilities, the dormitories, the kitchen, the school.

"Would it be possible," he asked, "for you to take Moïse in now?"

And that is what we did.

He lives there to this day, as does Chika's sister Mirlanda.

The world is an amazing place.

Let us end with this story. I used to drink coffee every morning. Chika would watch me make it, and, as was her way, she would coo, "What's *that*?"

"It's coffee, Chika."

"I wish *I* had some coffee."

She asked for months. The more I told her coffee wasn't for children, the more she wanted it. Finally, one morning, I relented, and she held the cup in both hands and took the smallest of sips and said, "Mmmmm!"

I still don't know if she really liked it, or just enjoyed feeling more grown-up.

And that, as we look back on things, is what haunts us the most. Not the struggle. Not the disease. The fact that the years pass and we say, "Chika would have been eight" or "Chika would have been nine," or, one day, "Chika would be in college now, drinking coffee." It's not the time she spent battling we lament. It's the growing up she missed. The time she didn't get. The future she never saw. That still seems so unfair.

But none of us are assured of tomorrow. It's what we do with today that makes an impact. Chika filled every day. She drank it in. She lived it up. And always, always, she affected someone, most often by making them smile.

People ask what I learned from this experience. I've tried in these pages to lay that out. But I can say one thing above all else. Families are like pieces of art, they can be made from many materials. Sometimes they are from birth, sometimes they are melded, sometimes they are merely time and circumstance mixing together, like eggs being scrambled in a Michigan kitchen.

But no matter how a family comes together, and no matter how it comes apart, this is true and will always be true: you cannot lose a child. And we did not lose a child. We were given one.

And she was glorious.

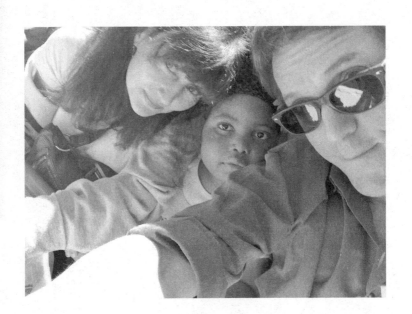

Acknowledgments

———

Seven years is far too short a life, but it is long enough to have touched—and be touched by—many others. I would like to give credit here to the people who touched Chika's brief but inspiring time on earth.

First, to those who nurtured her in health: our entire team at the Have Faith Haiti Orphanage—the nannies; the teachers; the support staff; our Haitian directors, Alain and Yonel; and our American directors, Jeff and Patty, Jennifer and Jeremiah, Anachemy, and Gina. Your dedication to Chika—and to all our children—is beyond inspiring.

Herzulia Desamour, Chika's godmother, took her in when Chika's mother died. Rolande St. Lot helped steer her to us. And her forty-plus Haitian brothers and sisters at the orphanage gave Chika someone to love and play with every minute of her time there.

Once her battle with DIPG began, the list grew longer. One life touches so many others. In no special order, thanks to all these people who helped along the way:

The incredible staff at C.S. Mott Children's Hospital in Ann Arbor, Michigan, who embraced Chika like a beacon of joyous light and helped defray the enormous costs of her care: Dr. Pat Robertson, Dr. Carl Koschmann, Dr. Hugh Garton, and Dr. Greg Thompson viewed Chika inside out, and the countless doctors, nurses, and support team always made her feel special during her hospital stays. No wonder there is a Superman in your lobby.

Equal thanks are due to Beaumont Hospital in Royal Oak, Michigan, and its incredible radiology team, led by Dr. Peter Chen. The staff there sent Chika home with more toys than a Walmart, and let her ring the bell when she finished her treatments. She hugged every one of you.

The team at Memorial Sloan Kettering in New York, under the dogged inspiration of Dr. Souweidane, deserves gratitude. We hope that information learned from Chika will benefit others trying the CED approach.

And in Germany, enormous thanks to Dr. Van Gool and the smart and kind staff at IOZK in Cologne. Chika was so happy during her time there. I think she sensed you are onto something right with immunology. And to the family and memory of little Gianna, who, however briefly, became Chika's overseas friend.

Special thanks to Tammi, Jason, and Lloyd Carr, who took their heartbreak and turned it into inspiring action with the Chad Tough Foundation. You did for us what we have tried to do for others climbing the DIPG mountain. Someday, thanks to folks like you, someone will get over the top.

Our endless gratitude to the many other organizations who embraced Chika: Walk the Line to SCI Recovery (Erica and Ira and the teams who came to our home); Health Partners, Inc. (John Prosser, Donna, and the incredible nurses who came through after midnight); all the folks at Hospice of Michigan and Dr. Ken Pituch and the team from Ann Arbor; Born Yoga in Birmingham, Michigan (thank you, Ashley, for letting Chika fly); and our homegrown house-call medical team of Judy, Jill, Susie, Mary, and "Dr." Michelle. To Julie Ford for teaching us PICC lines, Greg Holmes and Katherine Roth for their vast nutritional knowledge, Dr. Hunt for Chika's teeth, and Kevin and Cindy, for that special little chair.

And then there are Chika's "friends." Age meant nothing to her. Only your heart and your time. For sharing those so generously with our little girl, deepest thanks, in again, no special order, to Frank (who took her everywhere); Kim and Walid (who took her everywhere else); Nicole M. (Baba . . . ghan-*oush*!); Dianne (her admired teacher); Dr. Val and Rick (her favorite dog visits); Marina, Rudy and Chris (her Belgian hosts); Antoinetta (her Cologne host); Margareth, the Alley family and "Grandma" Peggy; "Pastor Donkey," Jordan, Lyn, Carmella, Catherine (swimming); Connie and Linda (who kept our house and us from falling apart many times); Dr. Chad Audi and family, Rosemary, Margie M., Terrie and Doug, Monica and Heath, Vito, Sandy, Taki, Yuki, Tomoko and Kaz, Perry G., Mike and Trish ("Silence!"), Della, Sara Werr, LaKema C.; and, of course, always, our extended loving family of Cara, my tireless, brilliant sister, who kept Chika's lessons coming; my brother

Acknowledgments

Peter, who made Chika laugh; Kathy, Tricia, and "Papa" Rick, Greg, Anne-Marie and sons (we all know how she felt about Aidan); Johnny S., and all our many nieces and nephews who knew her: Jesse and Marlee, Gabriel, Laura Beth, Nicole S., Johnny, Daniel, Michael and Lindsay, (little) Janine and Anton and daughters, Devon and Steven, Alex, David and Jenny, Paul, Joey and Josh.

Our family became her family, and she reveled in that.

My work world also melded into Chika's world, so deep thanks to "Mr. Marc" Rosenthal, "Mr. Mark" Mendelsohn (she never called you a bum), Kerri (for endless transcriptions), Jo-Ann, Vince, Antonella, my radio staff, Jean Yee and Lisa Goich (for showering Chika with kindness from afar), and the folks in my publishing world who showed great patience when I choose time with Chika over my work.

As for this book, it doesn't happen without David Black, who spent decades trying to tell me I would be a good father, and his wonderful team at Black, Inc., Susan Raihofer, Matt Belford, and Skyler Addison. My editor, Karen Rinaldi, wrestled with me like Jacob and the Angel, but only to get the best version of this story on paper, and I thank her very much for that. The rest of the fine folks at Harper have my humble appreciation: Jonathan Burnham, Leah Wasielewski, Stephanie Cooper, Doug Jones, Leslie Cohen, Tina Andreadis, Emily VanDerwerken, Jacqui Daniels, Rebecca Raskin, Hannah Robinson, Milan Bozic, Leah Carlson-Stanisic, John Jusino, Michael Siebert, and the many others who help to shepherd my book through to publication.

Acknowledgments

I wish to thank all our friends, colleagues, and doctors not listed individually here, because everyone who keeps you going on a journey like this, even for a day, becomes a small part of the story.

Finally, there is the largest part: Janine. During the year that I wrote this book, she would listen to me read the pages aloud, and it was hard and crushing and loving and exhilarating, which is what having a precious but sick child is like.

This is only my story because it was her story as well.

Chika. Janine. Me.

Us.

Mitch Albom
Detroit, Michigan
August 2019

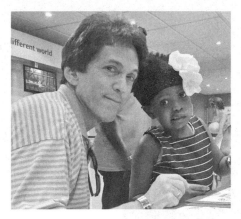

About the Author

MITCH ALBOM is the author of numerous works of fiction and nonfiction. He has written seven number one *New York Times* bestsellers, including *Tuesdays with Morrie*, the best-selling memoir of all time. His books have collectively sold more than forty million copies worldwide and have been translated into forty-seven languages in forty-nine territories. Albom has also penned award-winning TV films, internationally produced stage plays, a musical, and, for thirty years, a syndicated newspaper column. He was voted America's best sports columnist by the Associated Press Sports Editors thirteen times in his career. In 2006 Albom founded SAY Detroit, which now oversees nine full-time charities in the metro Detroit area, and in 2010 he began operating the Have Faith Haiti Orphanage in Port-au-Prince, which he visits monthly. He and his wife, Janine, live in Michigan.

All author profits from this book go to the
Have Faith Haiti Orphanage.